Obesity and Asthma

Editor

ANURAG AGRAWAL

IMMUNOLOGY AND ALLERGY CLINICS OF NORTH AMERICA

www.immunology.theclinics.com

Consulting Editor
RAFEUL ALAM

November 2014 • Volume 34 • Number 4

ELSEVIER

1600 John F. Kennedy Boulevard • Suite 1800 • Philadelphia, Pennsylvania, 19103-2899

http://www.theclinics.com

IMMUNOLOGY AND ALLERGY CLINICS OF NORTH AMERICA Volume 34, Number 4

November 2014 ISSN 0889–8561, ISBN-13: 978-0-323-32377-2

Editor: Jessica McCool

Developmental Editor: Stephanie Carter

Immunology and Allergy Clinics of North America (ISSN 0889–8561) is published quarterly by Elsevier Inc., 360 Park Avenue South, New York, NY 10010-1710. Months of issue are February, May, August, and November. Periodicals postage paid at New York, NY and additional mailing offices. Subscription prices are $320.00 per year for US individuals, $454.00 per year for US institutions, $150.00 per year for US students and residents, $395.00 per year for Canadian individuals, $220.00 per year for Canadian students, $577.00 per year for Canadian institutions, $445.00 per year for international individuals, $577.00 per year for international institutions, $220.00 per year for international students. To receive student/resident rate, orders must be accompanied by name of affiliated institution, date of term, and the *signature* of program/residency coordinator on institution letterhead. Orders will be billed at individual rate until proof of status is received. Foreign air speed delivery is included in all *Clinics* subscription prices. All prices are subject to change without notice. **POSTMASTER:** Send address changes to *Immunology and Allergy Clinics of North America,* Elsevier Health Sciences Division, Subscription Customer Service, 3251 Riverport Lane, Maryland Heights, MO 63043. **Customer Service: 1-800-654-2452 (U.S. and Canada); 314-447-8871 (outside U.S. and Canada). Fax: 314-447-8029. E-mail: journalscustomerservice-usa@elsevier.com (for print support); journalsonlinesupport-usa@elsevier.com (for online support).**

Reprints. For copies of 100 or more, of articles in this publication, please contact the Commercial Reprints Department, Elsevier Inc., 360 Park Avenue South, New York, New York 10010-1710. Tel. 212-633-3874, Fax: 212-633-3820, E-mail: reprints@elsevier.com.

Immunology and Allergy Clinics of North America is covered in MEDLINE/PubMed (Index Medicus), Current Contents/Life Sciences, Science Citation Index, ISI/BIOMED, Chemical Abstracts, and EMBASE/Excerpta Medica.

Contributors

CONSULTING EDITOR

RAFEUL ALAM, MD, PhD
Professor and Chief, Division of Allergy and Immunology, National Jewish Health, University of Colorado Denver, Denver, Colorado

EDITOR

ANURAG AGRAWAL, MD, PhD, FCCP
Molecular Immunogenetics Laboratory, Centre of Excellence for Translational Research in Asthma and Lung Disease, CSIR-Institute of Genomics and Integrative Biology, Delhi, India

AUTHORS

ANURAG AGRAWAL, MD, PhD, FCCP
Molecular Immunogenetics Laboratory, Centre of Excellence for Translational Research in Asthma and Lung Disease, CSIR-Institute of Genomics and Integrative Biology, Delhi, India

JENNIFER M. BRATT, PhD
Post-Doctoral Researcher, Division of Pulmonary, Critical Care and Sleep Medicine, Department of Internal Medicine, University of California, Davis, Davis, California

JEFFREY M. CRAIG, PhD
Associate Professor, Department of Paediatrics, Early Life Epigenetics Group, Murdoch Children's Research Institute, Royal Children's Hospital, University of Melbourne, Parkville, Victoria, Australia

JENNIFER DIAZ, MD
North Shore-Long Island Jewish Health System, Hofstra School of Medicine, Great Neck, New York

SHERRY FARZAN, MD
North Shore-Long Island Jewish Health System, Hofstra School of Medicine, Great Neck, New York

HARTMUT GRASEMANN, MD, PhD
Program in Physiology and Experimental Medicine, Research Institute, Division of Respiratory Medicine, Department of Pediatrics, The Hospital for Sick Children, University of Toronto, Toronto, Ontario, Canada

TIMOTHY HEACOCK, MD
Department of Pulmonary and Critical Care, Duke University Medical Center, Durham, North Carolina

RAE-CHI HUANG, MD, PhD
Associate Professor, Members of '*In-FLAME*' the International Inflammation Network, World Universities Network (WUN); Telethon KIDS Institute, University of Western Australia, Subiaco, Western Australia, Australia

SUSHIL K. KABRA, MD
Professor, Department of Pediatrics, All India Institute of Medical Sciences, Ansari Nagar, New Delhi, India

NICHOLAS J. KENYON, MD, MAS
Professor, Division of Pulmonary, Critical Care and Sleep Medicine, Department of Internal Medicine, University of California, Davis, Davis, California

SNEHA LIMAYE, MBBS, PDCR
Head of Department-Clinical Trials, Chest Research Foundation, Pune, India

ANGELA L. LINDERHOLM, PhD
Assistant Project Scientist, Division of Pulmonary, Critical Care and Sleep Medicine, Department of Internal Medicine, University of California, Davis, Davis, California

RAKESH LODHA, MD
Additional Professor, Department of Pediatrics, All India Institute of Medical Sciences, Ansari Nagar, New Delhi, India

NJIRA LUGOGO, MD
Assistant Professor of Medicine, Department of Pulmonary and Critical Care, Duke University Medical Center, Durham, North Carolina

DEBRA J. PALMER, PhD
Associate Professor, School of Paediatrics and Child Health, University of Western Australia (M561), Subiaco, Western Australia, Australia; Members of '*In-FLAME*' the International Inflammation Network, World Universities Network (WUN)

MIRIAM K. PEREZ, MD
Associate Staff, Pediatric Institute and Children's Hospital, Cleveland Clinic, Cleveland, Ohio

GIOVANNI PIEDIMONTE, MD
Professor and Chairman, Pediatric Institute; Physician-in-Chief, Children's Hospital; President, Children's Hospital for Rehabilitation, Cleveland Clinic, Cleveland, Ohio

Y.S. PRAKASH, MD, PhD
Departments of Anesthesiology and Physiology and Biomedical Engineering, Mayo Clinic, Rochester, Minnesota

SUSAN L. PRESCOTT, MD, PhD
Professor, School of Paediatrics and Child Health, University of Western Australia (M561), Subiaco, Western Australia, Australia; Members of '*In-FLAME*' the International Inflammation Network, World Universities Network (WUN); Telethon KIDS Institute, University of Western Australia, Subiaco, Western Australia, Australia

DINESH RAJ, MD
Consultant, Department of Pediatrics, Holy Family Hospital, Okhla, New Delhi, India

SUNDEEP SALVI, MD, DNB, PhD(UK), FCCP (USA)
Director, Chest Research Foundation, Pune, India

GERTRUD U. SCHUSTER, PhD
Assistant Project Scientist, Nutrition Department, University of California, Davis;
Immunity and Diseases Prevention Unit, Western Human Nutrition Research Center,
United States Department of Agriculture (USDA), Agricultural Research Services (ARS),
Davis, California

JEREMY A. SCOTT, PhD
Division of Biomedical Sciences, Department of Health Sciences, Faculty of Health
and Behavioural Sciences, Northern Ontario School of Medicine, Lakehead University,
Thunder Bay, Ontario, Canada

AMIR A. ZEKI, MD, MAS
Assistant Professor, Division of Pulmonary, Critical Care and Sleep Medicine, Department
of Internal Medicine, University of California, Davis, Davis, California

Contents

The concomitant increase in obesity and asthma in recent years has led to the classification of two obese-asthma phenotypes, characterized by the age of asthma onset and atopy. Asthma tends to be more severe, harder to control, and more resistant to standard medications among members of these two groups. Because of the limited effectiveness of inhaled corticosteroids, dietary changes and weight loss measures must be considered in the management of these patients. Furthermore, comorbidities such as depression and obstructive sleep apnea must be addressed to provide optimal care for this group of difficult-to-control asthmatics.

The simultaneous increment in the prevalence of obesity and allergic diseases suggests a possible link between them. This review focuses on the consequences of obesity on allergic diseases, especially asthma in children and adolescents, and evaluates the available evidence on the possible mechanisms. Obesity is related more strongly to nonatopic than atopic asthma, suggesting non-eosinophilic inflammation and Th1 polarization. Among other allergic diseases, the association is more consistent with eczema compared to allergic rhinitis/rhinoconjunctivitis. The mechanisms of asthma in obese individuals could involve mechanical effects of obesity on lung function, adipokines-mediated inflammation, shared factors (diet, genetics, sedentary lifestyle) and comorbidities.

Nitric oxide (NO) is important in the regulation of airway tone and airway responsiveness. Alterations in the L-arginine metabolism resulting in reduced availability of the substrate L-arginine for NO synthases, as well as the presence of NO synthase inhibitors such as asymmetric dimethylarginine, contribute to the reduced NO formation and airway dysfunction in asthma. Therapeutic interventions aiming to modulate the impaired L-arginine metabolism may help correct the enhanced airway tone and responsiveness in asthma.

Childhood asthma and obesity have reached epidemic proportions worldwide, and the latter is also contributing to increasing rates of related metabolic disorders, such as diabetes. However, the relationship between asthma, obesity, and abnormal metabolism is not well understood nor has it been adequately explored in children. This article discusses the concept of metabolic asthma and the recent hypothesis that early derangement in lipid and glucose metabolism is independently associated with increased risk for asthma.

Multiple studies have determined that obesity increases asthma risk or severity. Metabolic changes of obesity, such as diabetes or insulin resistance, are associated with asthma and poorer lung function. Insulin resistance is also found to increase asthma risk independent of body mass. Conversely, asthma is associated with abnormal glucose and lipid metabolism, insulin resistance, and obesity. Here we review our current understanding of how dietary and lifestyle factors lead to changes in mitochondrial metabolism and cellular bioenergetics, inducing various components of the cardiometabolic syndrome and airway disease.

Obesity and asthma have increasingly been linked with an increased risk of developing asthma associated with increasing body mass index. Overweight/obese patients with asthma have more symptoms, poor asthma control, and decreased response to conventional asthma therapies. Weight loss may be associated with improvements in asthma control, response to medications, and overall asthma-related quality of life. This article discusses the effect of weight loss via dietary modifications and surgical interventions on asthma symptoms and control. Weight loss should be encouraged as a means of improving asthma control but there are insufficient data to recommend surgical interventions solely for this purpose.

Asthma is a complex syndrome that affects an estimated 26 million people in the United States but gaps exist in the recognition and management of asthmatic subgroups. This article proposes alternative approaches for future treatments of adult obese asthmatics who do not respond to standard controller therapies, drawing parallels between seemingly disparate therapeutics through their common signaling pathways. How metformin and statins can potentially improve airway inflammation is described and supplements are suggested. A move toward more targeted therapies for asthma subgroups is needed. These therapies address asthma and the comorbidities that accompany obesity and metabolic syndrome to provide the greatest therapeutic potential.

Observational studies show consistent links between early-life nutritional exposures as important risk factors for the development of asthma, allergy, and obesity. Reliance on increasing use of dietary supplementation and fortification (eg, with folate) to compensate for increased consumption of processed foods is also influencing immune and metabolic outcomes. Epigenetics is providing substantial advances in understanding how early-life nutritional exposures can effect disease development. This article summarizes current evidence linking the influence of early-life nutritional exposures on epigenetic regulation with a focus on the disease outcomes of asthma, allergy, and obesity.

Air pollution is a well-known risk for lung diseases, including asthma. Growing evidences suggesting air pollution as a novel risk factor for the development of obesity. Several Epidemiological studies have ascertained an association between various ambient and indoor air pollutants and obesity by medium of endocrine disruptive chemicals that can disrupt the normal development and homeostatic controls over adipogenesis and energy balance and induce obesity. Several obesity-induced mechanisms have been proposed that increases this vulnerability of obese individuals to harmful effects of air pollution rendering them more susceptible to developing air-pollution driven incident asthma or worsening of already existing asthma.

IMMUNOLOGY AND ALLERGY CLINICS OF NORTH AMERICA

FORTHCOMING ISSUES

February 2015
Pediatric Allergy
Robert Wood,
Pamela Frischmeyer-Guerrerio,
and Corinne Keet, *Editors*

May 2015
Anaphylaxis
Anne Marie Ditto, *Editor*

August 2015
Eosinophil-Associated Disorders
Amy D. Klion and Princess Ogbogu,
Editors

RECENT ISSUES

August 2014
Drug Hypersensitivity
Pascal Demoly, *Editor*

May 2014
Mastocytosis
Cem Akin, *Editor*

February 2014
Urticaria
Malcolm Greaves, *Editor*

ISSUE OF RELATED INTEREST

Clinics in Chest Medicine, March 2014 (Vol. 35, Issue 1)
Chronic Obstructive Pulmonary Disease
Peter J. Barnes, *Editor*
http://www.chestmed.theclinics.com/

NOW AVAILABLE FOR YOUR iPhone and iPad

Foreword

Obesity and Asthma—Is There a Causal Association?

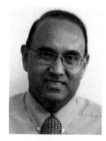

Rafeul Alam, MD, PhD
Consulting Editor

The increase in obesity is a worldwide problem. Obesity does not specifically affect asthma. It affects many chronic illnesses. Our challenge is to understand how obesity contributes to allergy and asthma. Obesity can directly affect lung function, which is mostly restrictive in nature. Distal lung compliance is preferentially affected in obese asthmatic patients, which could, in part, explain the mechanical aspect of obesity-induced asthma.[1] How it affects airway obstruction is the question. There are many potential factors that could contribute to this condition. Increased BMI, abdominal obesity, metabolic syndrome, obesity-associated inflammation—all of these factors could work independently or in concert. There are controversies about obesity-associated asthma and Th2/eosinophilic inflammation. Peripheral low eosinophils and exhaled nitric oxide have been reported to be low in obese asthmatic patients.[2] This has been interpreted as an indication of a non-Th2 mechanism of obesity-associated asthma. However, a recent bronchial biopsy study demonstrated a select increase in eosinophils in the airway mucosa in obese asthmatic patients.[3] Thus, the association and mechanistic connection between obesity and Th2 inflammation requires additional studies. The role of type 2 innate lymphoid in obesity-associated asthma is currently unknown. It is interesting to note that eosinophils and Th2 cytokines prevent adipogenesis in mice and favor beige fat development, which prevents obesity. This paradigm does not appear to work in human asthma.[4] Animal studies imply a role of type 3 innate lymphoid cells producing IL17A in obesity-induced asthma.[5]

Dietary fiber affects gut microbiota, increases short chain fatty acid production, and consequently inhibits allergic inflammation in the airways.[6] Since obesity frequently results from consumption of high-caloric-containing and low-fiber-containing foods, our

---

Supported by National Institutes of Health Grants RO1 AI091614, AI102943, and N01 HHSN272200700048C.

Immunol Allergy Clin N Am 34 (2014) xi–xii
http://dx.doi.org/10.1016/j.iac.2014.09.001
immunology.theclinics.com

food preferences could set the stage for simultaneous and parallel development of obesity and asthma. Recent studies suggest that subcellular organelle (eg, mitochondria, endoplasmic reticulum) dysfunction could trigger biochemical alterations resulting in insulin resistance, metabolic syndrome, obesity, and asthma.

Given its growing prevalence, obesity is likely to become an important feature of asthma phenotype. We need basic science research to fully understand its pathogenesis. We need clinical studies to prevent and better manage this condition. To update us on this important field of research, Dr Anurag Agrawal, a leader in the field, has brought together an outstanding group of experts covering epidemiologic, mechanistic, and clinical aspects of obesity-associated asthma.

Rafeul Alam, MD, PhD
Division of Allergy and Immunology
National Jewish Health
University of Colorado Denver School of Medicine
1400 Jackson Street
Denver, CO 80206, USA

E-mail address:
alamr@njhealth.org

REFERENCES

1. Al-Alwan A, Bates JH, Chapman DG, et al. The nonallergic asthma of obesity. A matter of distal lung compliance. Am J Respir Crit Care Med 2014;189(12): 1494–502.
2. Sutherland ER, Goleva E, King TS, et al. Asthma Clinical Research Network. Cluster analysis of obesity and asthma phenotypes. PLoS One 2012;7(5):e36631.
3. Desai D, Newby C, Symon FA, et al. Elevated sputum interleukin-5 and submucosal eosinophilia in obese individuals with severe asthma. Am J Respir Crit Care Med 2013;188(6):657–63.
4. Qiu Y, Nguyen KD, Odegaard JI, et al. Eosinophils and type 2 cytokine signaling in macrophages orchestrate development of functional beige fat. Cell 2014; 157(6):1292–308.
5. Kim HY, Lee HJ, Chang YJ, et al. Interleukin-17-producing innate lymphoid cells and the NLRP3 inflammasome facilitate obesity-associated airway hyperreactivity. Nat Med 2014;20(1):54–61.
6. Trompette A, Gollwitzer ES, Yadava K, et al. Gut microbiota metabolism of dietary fiber influences allergic airway disease and hematopoiesis. Nat Med 2014;20(2): 159–66.

Preface

Urban, Obese, Allergic, and Breathless: The Shape of Things to Come?

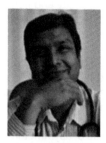

Anurag Agrawal, MD, PhD, FCCP
Editor

There has been a paradigm shift in lifestyle and availability of food over the last century that has inverted the health challenges to society. Once the rich were fat, the poor were thin, putting food on the table was a challenge, and communicable infectious diseases were the biggest threats. While this continues in the less-developed world, elsewhere the rich are thin, the poor are fat, and obesity is a major health challenge along with associated noncommunicable diseases. Increasing availability of inexpensive food, reduced necessity of manual work, growth of sedentary recreational activities, and limited access to active lifestyles has driven this change. Beyond the expected increase in well-known obesity-associated diseases like diabetes and cardiovascular disease, this global epidemic of obesity has also been mirrored by equally large increases in asthma.[1,2] These twin epidemics of asthma and obesity are strongly correlated epidemiologically, and the mechanistic links are also becoming increasingly clear.[3–5] This special issue is devoted to providing the reader with an understanding of why asthma and obesity are on the rise, the magnitude and mechanism of increased asthma risk in obese subjects, the different clinical profile of asthmatic patients with concomitant obesity, and finally, the proven and expected benefits of adjunct therapies targeting weight loss and/or metabolic function in such patients.

The concept of "obese-asthma" as a new subphenotype of asthma is important for practicing clinicians. Many practices have already seen a shift from the typical asthma patient of the past who started experiencing symptoms early in life and had a strong allergic component to those starting much later in life and without obvious allergic triggers. Such patients are often female and obese and represent a form of obese-asthma.[5–7] This is an important clinical subphenotype because such patients tend to have high symptoms but little allergic inflammation, as measured by exhaled nitric oxide (exhNO) or sputum eosinophils, and tend to respond poorly to standard

Immunol Allergy Clin N Am 34 (2014) xiii–xviii
http://dx.doi.org/10.1016/j.iac.2014.07.010
0889-8561/14/$ – see front matter
immunology.theclinics.com

anti-inflammatory therapy, including corticosteroids. It should be noted that exhNO could be an unreliable marker in obese subjects, as discussed subsequently. There are also a substantial number of obese-asthmatics with early-onset asthma and strong allergic component, who require more intensive anti-inflammatory therapy. In this issue, Sherry Farzan and Jennifer Diaz review the clinical implications of the adult obese-asthma phenotypes and highlight the challenges that they pose.

In children, obesity has been strongly associated with asthma but not with other allergic diseases. Rakesh Lodha and colleagues review the available data from child-hood studies and find consistent strong associations between obesity and nonatopic asthma but not between obesity and atopic-asthma or other allergic diseases. This challenges experimental models of obese-asthma, where adipose-hormone–mediated inflammation augments Th2 inflammation and the allergic response. It re-mains possible, however, that adipose hormones have lung-specific effects rather than a general potentiation of allergy. Other important possibilities include induction of asthma-like features by metabolic changes of obesity. Nitric oxide (NO) is important in the regulation of airway tone and airway responsiveness, and NO metabolism has been reported to be abnormal in obese subjects with metabolic syndrome.[4,8,9] Reduced availability of the substrate L-arginine and the presence of asymmetric dime-thylarginine (ADMA), an uncoupler of NO synthases, contributes to reduced NO forma-tion, increased superoxide generation, and increased smooth muscle tone in obesity, metabolic syndrome, and asthma.[10–14] This also sheds light on why exhaled NO, used clinically as a marker for eosinophilic inflammation, is diminished in obese asthmatics. In this issue, Hartmut Grasemann and Jeremy Scott review the current understanding of the role of ADMA in asthma pathogenesis and conclude that ADMA may represent a novel therapeutic target in correcting the enhanced airways responsiveness in asthma. Others and we have previously proposed a role for hyperinsulinemia in pro-moting airway hyperresponsiveness (AHR) and remodeling.[15,16] Insulin promotes airway smooth muscle proliferation and contractility and can also lead to extracellular matrix deposition by fibroblasts. These changes can remodel the airways and lead to AHR independent of inflammation. Insulin resistance (IR) was indeed found be a stron-ger predictor of aeroallergen sensitization and asthma than obesity in a Danish cohort, but this has not been consistently seen.[17,18] This has been reviewed in more detail elsewhere.[16] Interestingly, not only are IR and consequent hyperinsulinemia well known in obesity, but also markers of IR, such as acanthosis nigricans and dyslipide-mia, have been noted in asthmatic children.[19] Giovanni Piedimonte and Miriam Perez review the current data on metabolic consequences of asthma to bring out the con-nections between asthma, obesity, and diabetes.

While IR appears to be one of the important functional threads running through obesity and asthma, there appear to be deeper mechanistic links. At a subcellular level, development of IR has been related to mitochondrial dysfunction and increased mitochondrial reactive oxygen species generation.[20] This, together with endoplasmic reticulum stress, represents an emerging interface between obesity, metabolic syn-drome, and airway disease, which can be triggered by nutrient overload, inflammation, or cigarette smoke, among others.[21–26] Unpublished data from our lab suggest that high-fat-diet–induced obesity or high-sugar-diet–induced IR and hyperinsulinemia are both related to ER stress and mitochondrial dysfunction. Spontaneous AHR and remodeling are seen in such mice without any allergic inflammation and also the allergic response is augmented. In this issue, YS Prakash and I review the concept of obesity and asthma as diseases of bioenergetic failure and mitochondrial dysfunc-tion. In support, mitochondrial transfer from mesenchymal stem cells (MSC) strongly attenuates allergic asthma in mice.[23] The effect is clearly related to mitochondrial transfer because MSC lacking mitochondrial transfer capacity are ineffective, while those that are bioengineered for greater mitochondrial donor potential are much more effective.[27] We believe that bioenergetic failure is a common theme between multiple metabolic and cardiopulmonary disorders and merits further examination as a therapeutic target.[24,28] Possible interventions to improve mitochondrial health are discussed in the review with the expectation that these may have benefit in asthma. Of these, Coenzyme Q10 supplementation has been reported to be potentially beneficial in steroid-resistant asthmatics.[29,30] Benefit in obese-asthma remains to be tested.

Current guidelines for the management of asthma do not recognize obesity as a guiding factor in determining optimal therapy. Since obese asthmatics do not respond as well to the recommended standard controller therapies as normal-weight persons, this is a critical gap in the recognition and management of an important subgroup. This issue has two important reviews that address this gap and provide information to the reader regarding additional options for poorly controlled severe asthma patients, who are also obese. First, since many of the mechanisms of pathogenesis of asthma relate to metabolic consequences of caloric excess, adiposity, and adipose hormones, it is intuitive that caloric restriction and weight loss should be recommended. However, this does not work for all patients, and evidence of substantial benefit is required for initiation of therapeutic programs beyond counseling. Njira Lugogo and Timothy Heacock review the evidence for medical or surgical weight loss strategies in the management of obese-asthma and conclude that weight loss should be encouraged as a means of improving asthma symptoms and control, but there are insufficient data to recommend surgical interventions for weight loss solely for the purpose of improving asthma.

Second, other than nutritional and lifestyle modification, there may be an additional role for drugs and/or supplements that target the principal pathological abnormalities. Statins and metformin have been found to be effective agents for the treatment of asthma in animal models and are also suitable for the treatment of obesity-associated metabolic dysfunction.[4,31–33] Metformin, in particular, has been associated with attenuation of the augmented allergic inflammation in obese mice on a high-fat diet. One of the mechanisms by which statins work seems to be induction of dimethylarginine dimethylamino hydrolase1 and inhibition of arginase, thereby resulting in an increased ratio of L-arginine/ADMA, thereby increasing L-arginine bioavailability to NOS.[34,35] In an alternate approach, L-arginine supplementation at high doses is similarly effective, probably by restoring a normal L-arginine/ADMA ratio, overcoming the uncoupling effects of high ADMA and promoting NO synthesis.[36–38] There are some concerns, however, on whether increased arginase-mediated degradation of L-arginine may worsen asthma and simultaneous arginase inhibition may be required.[38] Nicholas Kenyon and colleagues review the current data on such novel therapies targeting asthma and the comorbidities that accompany obesity. In their severe asthma clinics, they have found that female-predominant severe asthmatics with a mean body mass index of 30 or more, benefited from statin treatment. They are also currently testing the benefit of L-arginine supplementation in severe asthmatics, who are predominantly overweight/obese and female. Nutritional supplements like L-arginine and omega-3 fatty acids are other exciting considerations for future treatment of asthma that may additionally attenuate the metabolic syndrome. Overall, there is a pressing need for greater recognition of the obese-asthma subtypes and a move toward more targeted therapies.

Notwithstanding any of the mechanisms by which obesity leads to asthma and the many possible therapeutic strategies for obese-asthma, it seems certain that the twin epidemics of asthma relate mostly to external modifiable factors. Given that an ounce of prevention is better than a pound of cure, we must also focus on the underlying risks that are driving both obesity and asthma. Since rapid increases in obesity and asthma have been seen in childhood, this requires consideration of prenatal and postnatal factors. In particular, calorie-rich but nutrition-poor food products and environmental pollution are modifiable social risks that retard the development of our lungs even before we are born and accelerate the decline thereafter. In this issue, Debra Palmer and colleagues along with Sundeep Salvi and Sneha Limaye shed light on this poorly understood facet in both of their articles. It emerges that protection of the nutrition of young women and provision of a clean environment are time-critical interventions that cannot be delayed further. However, more is not always better, whether calories or supplements! For example, maternal folate supplementation in late pregnancy, when the risk for neural tube defects has already passed, has been associated with increased risk of allergy and asthma.[39] Could this prevalent practice be altering the epigenome and driving the ever higher peaks in the prevalence of these diseases?

It is time to heed the eloquent call by Giovanni Piedimonte and Miriam Perez in this issue, "If we want to prevail in the war against chronic airway diseases that so far have eluded any therapeutic strategy, it is essential to recognize that the months spent in our mother's womb may be the most consequential of our lives, and identify the intrauterine and early life events shaping the development of the respiratory system to prevent or redirect dysfunctional phenotypes before they result in actual disease." This emphasized, I encourage you to enjoy the expert reviews in this special issue that explore each of these aspects in greater detail.

ACKNOWLEDGMENTS

Anurag Agrawal is supported by the Lady Tata Memorial Trust and the CSIR Center of Excellence for Translational Research in Asthma and Lung Disease.

Anurag Agrawal, MD, PhD, FCCP
Centre of Excellence for Translational Research
in Asthma and Lung Disease
CSIR–Institute of Genomics and
Integrative Biology
Mall Road
Delhi 110007, India

E-mail address:
a.agrawal@igib.in

REFERENCES

1. Kent BD, Lane SJ. Twin epidemics: asthma and obesity. Int Arch Allergy Immunol 2012;157(3):213–4.
2. Beuther DA. Recent insight into obesity and asthma. Curr Opin Pulm Med 2010; 16(1):64–70.
3. Agrawal A, Sood A, Linneberg A, et al. Mechanistic understanding of the effect of obesity on asthma and allergy. J Allergy 2013;2013:598904.
4. Agrawal A, Mabalirajan U, Ahmad T, et al. Emerging interface between metabolic syndrome and asthma. Am J Respir Cell Mol Biol 2011;44(3):270–5.
5. Wenzel SE. Asthma phenotypes: the evolution from clinical to molecular approaches. Nat Med 2012;18(5):716–25.

6. Haldar P, Pavord ID, Shaw DE, et al. Cluster analysis and clinical asthma phenotypes. Am J Respir Crit Care Med 2008;178(3):218–24.
7. Fajt ML, Wenzel SE. Asthma phenotypes in adults and clinical implications. Expert Rev Respir Med 2009;3(6):607–25.
8. Puchau B, Zulet MA, Urtiaga G, et al. Asymmetric dimethylarginine association with antioxidants intake in healthy young adults: a role as an indicator of metabolic syndrome features. Metabolism 2009;58(10):1483–8.
9. Holguin F. Arginine and nitric oxide pathways in obesity-associated asthma. J Allergy 2013;2013:714595.
10. Carraro S, Giordano G, Piacentini G, et al. Asymmetric dimethylarginine in exhaled breath condensate and serum of children with asthma. Chest 2013; 144(2):405–10.
11. Holguin F, Comhair SA, Hazen SL, et al. An association between L-arginine/asymmetric dimethyl arginine balance, obesity, and the age of asthma onset phenotype. Am J Respir Crit Care Med 2013;187(2):153–9.
12. Scott JA, North ML, Rafii M, et al. Asymmetric dimethylarginine is increased in asthma. Am J Respir Crit Care Med 2011;184(7):779–85.
13. Ahmad T, Mabalirajan U, Sharma A, et al. Simvastatin improves epithelial dysfunction and airway hyperresponsiveness: from ADMA to asthma. Am J Respir Cell Mol Biol 2011;44(4):531–9.
14. Ahmad T, Mabalirajan U, Ghosh B, et al. Altered asymmetric dimethyl arginine metabolism in allergically inflamed mouse lungs. Am J Respir Cell Mol Biol 2010;42(1):3–8.
15. Nie Z, Jacoby DB, Fryer AD. Hyperinsulinemia potentiates airway responsiveness to parasympathetic nerve stimulation in obese rats. Am J Respir Cell Mol Biol 2014.
16. Singh S, Prakash YS, Linneberg A, et al. Insulin and the lung: connecting asthma and metabolic syndrome. J Allergy 2013;2013:627384.
17. Ma J, Xiao L, Knowles SB. Obesity, insulin resistance and the prevalence of atopy and asthma in US adults. Allergy 2010;65(11):1455–63.
18. Husemoen LL, Glumer C, Lau C, et al. Association of obesity and insulin resistance with asthma and aeroallergen sensitization. Allergy 2008;63(5):575–82.
19. Cottrell L, Neal WA, Ice C, et al. Metabolic abnormalities in children with asthma. Am J Respir Crit Care Med 2011;183(4):441–8.
20. Martin SD, McGee SL. The role of mitochondria in the aetiology of insulin resistance and type 2 diabetes. Biochim Biophys Acta 2014;1840(4):1303–12.
21. Makhija L, Krishnan V, Rehman R, et al. Chemical chaperones mitigate experimental asthma by attenuating endoplasmic reticulum stress. Am J Respir Cell Mol Biol 2014;50(5):923–31.
22. Aravamudan B, Kiel A, Freeman M, et al. Cigarette smoke-induced mitochondrial fragmentation and dysfunction in human airway smooth muscle. Am J Physiol Lung Cell Mol Physiol 2014;306(9):L840–54.
23. Ahmad T, Mukherjee S, Pattnaik B, et al. Miro1 regulates intercellular mitochondrial transport and enhances mesenchymal stem cell rescue efficacy. EMBO J 2014;33(9):994–1010.
24. Mabalirajan U, Ghosh B. Mitochondrial dysfunction in metabolic syndrome and asthma. J Allergy 2013;2013:340476.
25. Aguilera-Aguirre L, Bacsi A, Saavedra-Molina A, et al. Mitochondrial dysfunction increases allergic airway inflammation. J Immunol 2009;183(8):5379–87.
26. Mabalirajan U, Dinda AK, Kumar S, et al. Mitochondrial structural changes and dysfunction are associated with experimental allergic asthma. J Immunol 2008; 181(5):3540–8.

27. Las G, Shirihai OS. Miro1: New wheels for transferring mitochondria. EMBO J 2014;33(9):939–41.
28. Aravamudan B, Thompson MA, Pabelick CM, et al. Mitochondria in lung diseases. Expert Rev Respir Med 2013;7(6):631–46.
29. Gvozdjakova A, Kucharska J, Bartkovjakova M, et al. Coenzyme Q10 supplementation reduces corticosteroids dosage in patients with bronchial asthma. Biofactors 2005;25(1–4):235–40.
30. Gazdik F, Gvozdjakova A, Horvathova M, et al. Levels of coenzyme Q10 in asthmatics. Bratisl Lek Listy 2002;103(10):353–6.
31. Ahmad T, Mabalirajan U, Sharma A, et al. Simvastatin improves epithelial dysfunction and airway hyperresponsiveness: from asymmetric dimethyl-arginine to asthma. Am J Respir Cell Mol Biol 2011;44(4):531–9.
32. Calixto MC, Lintomen L, Andre DM, et al. Metformin attenuates the exacerbation of the allergic eosinophilic inflammation in high fat-diet-induced obesity in mice. PLoS One 2013;8(10):e76786.
33. Park CS, Bang BR, Kwon HS, et al. Metformin reduces airway inflammation and remodeling via activation of AMP-activated protein kinase. Biochem Pharmacol 2012;84(12):1660–70.
34. Kinker KG, Gibson AM, Bass SA, et al. Overexpression of dimethylarginine dimethylaminohydrolase 1 attenuates airway inflammation in a mouse model of asthma. PLoS One 2014;9(1):e85148.
35. Zeki AA, Bratt JM, Rabowsky M, et al. Simvastatin inhibits goblet cell hyperplasia and lung arginase in a mouse model of allergic asthma: a novel treatment for airway remodeling? Transl Res 2010;156(6):335–49.
36. Mabalirajan U, Ahmad T, Leishangthem GD, et al. L-arginine reduces mitochondrial dysfunction and airway injury in murine allergic airway inflammation. Int Immunopharmacol 2010;10(12):1514–9.
37. Mabalirajan U, Ahmad T, Leishangthem G, et al. Beneficial effects of high dose of L-arginine on airway hyperresponsiveness and airway inflammation in a murine model of asthma. J Allergy Clin Immunol 2010;125(3):626–35.
38. Bratt JM, Zeki AA, Last JA, et al. Competitive metabolism of L-arginine: arginase as a therapeutic target in asthma. J Biomed Res 2011;25(5):299–308.
39. Whitrow MJ, Moore VM, Rumbold AR, et al. Effect of supplemental folic acid in pregnancy on childhood asthma: a prospective birth cohort study. Am J Epidemiol 2009;170(12):1486–93.

Clinical Implications of the Obese-Asthma Phenotypes

Jennifer Diaz, MD, Sherry Farzan, MD*

KEYWORDS

- Obesity • Asthma • Phenotypes • Body mass index

KEY POINTS

- The prevalence of obesity and asthma around the world is increasing, and together they have led to the classification of two obese-asthma phenotypes.
- The two obese-asthma phenotypes are early-onset asthma, which has an atopic quality, and late-onset asthma, with less atopic features.
- Both obese-asthma phenotypes are characterized by a severe form of asthma, with more exacerbations and poorer symptom control compared with lean asthmatics.
- The obese-asthma phenotypes are less responsive to inhaled corticosteroid and therefore new avenues for treatment should be considered, including dietary changes, weight loss, and use of nonstandard medications.
- Comorbid conditions, such as depression and obstructive sleep apnea, must be addressed as complicating factors in asthma management.

INTRODUCTION

Across the United States and the world there is an large increase in the prevalence of both obesity and asthma. The burgeoning rates of these two epidemics are occurring in the both the adult and pediatric populations. With the increased incidence of obesity and asthma, new asthma phenotypes have emerged with different characteristics, presentation, and treatment responses compared with traditionally described asthma. This article discusses these evolving obese-asthma phenotypes.

EPIDEMIOLOGY
The Obesity Epidemic

An epidemic is defined as an outbreak or product of sudden rapid spread, growth, or development, usually used in health care to describe the spread of diseases.

Disclosure: S. Farzan has received research support from the Thrasher Foundation Award # 9174, New York State Empire Clinical Investigators Program, and Merck Study #39377. J. Diaz has nothing to disclose.
North Shore-Long Island Jewish Health System, Division of Allergy and Immunology, Hofstra School of Medicine, 865 Northern Boulevard, Suite 101, Great Neck, NY 11021, USA
* Corresponding author.
E-mail address: sfarzan@nshs.edu

Immunol Allergy Clin N Am 34 (2014) 739–751
http://dx.doi.org/10.1016/j.iac.2014.07.008
0889-8561/14/$ – see front matter © 2014 Elsevier Inc. All rights reserved.

However, because of its large increase in prevalence, obesity has reached epidemic status.

Obesity is classified using the body mass index (BMI) (**Table 1**). Some studies use waist circumference or percentage of body fat to determine weight classification, and this may be a better predictor of obesity-associated morbidity.[1–3]

According to a 2008 World Health Organization survey, more than half a billion adults around the world were categorized as being obese, and more than 1.4 billion were overweight, constituting 10% of the adult population.[4] More alarming findings exist in the United States, with the 2010 US Centers for Disease Control and Prevention (CDC) National Health and Nutrition Examination Survey (NHANES) showing more than 70 million adults and 12 million children (36% and 15%, respectively) considered obese.[5] With the increase of obesity in the United States has come an increase in heart disease and diabetes, as well as many other diseases, including asthma.

Asthma, Asthma Everywhere

The prevalence of asthma is also increasing. In the 2000 Behavior Risk Factor Surveillance Survey (BRFSS), most states reported an asthma prevalence of less than 8.3%. By the 2010 BRFSS, 46 states reported an asthma prevalence of greater than 11.5%.[6] According to a 2011 CDC health survey, 18.9 million adults (8.2%) and 7.1 million children (9.5%) in the United States were diagnosed with asthma. These numbers have increased by 4.3 million since 2001. Along with increasing prevalence have come increases in asthma-related medical costs, office/emergency room visits, and morbidity.[7] Therefore, it is important for clinicians to be able to recognize modifiable risk factors for development of severe asthma, such as obesity.

RISK FACTORS
Obesity and Asthma: Are These Related?

With the increase in prevalence of both asthma and obesity, it is crucial to examine the underlying relationship. Over the last decade there have been numerous studies showing that both obese adults and children are at a significantly higher risk of developing asthma.[3,8–10]

Pediatric population

Rodriguez and colleagues[9] examined NHANES data from more than 12,000 children and adolescents in an attempt to identify risk factors for pediatric asthma. Children and adolescents with a sex-specific BMI of greater than the 85th percentile had an almost 2-fold increased risk for developing asthma, which was more severe and difficult to control. Compared with other groups with similar risk factors (including parental

Table 1 Weight classification based on BMI	
Classification	**BMI (kg/m^2)**
Underweight	<18.5
Normal	18.5–24.9
Overweight	25–29.9
Obese (class 1)	30–34.9
Obese (class 2)	35–39.9
Extremely obese (class 3)	≥40

atopy), those with a higher BMI had more episodes of wheezing and hospitalizations. The timing of the weight gain plays a role in a child's level of risk for developing asthma. Children who gain an excessive amount of weight over the first 6 years of life, especially during infancy, are at an even higher risk for asthma than children who gain weight later in childhood.[11]

Adult population

The adult population shows a similar association between obesity and asthma. A meta-analysis including more than 300,000 subjects reported a 50% increase in the risk of developing asthma if the patient was obese or overweight. Among overweight individuals, the odds ratio of developing asthma was 1.32, whereas for obese individuals it was 1.92, showing a dose-response relationship between BMI and the risk of developing asthma. Similar to the pediatric population, obese asthmatics tend to develop a more severe, refractory form of asthma.[12,13] In the adult population, it has been argued that central obesity is predictive of only nonatopic asthma.[3] Published data reveal that 50% of asthmatics are obese, although it has not been established that asthma leads to obesity.[14]

Gender, race, and ethnicity

In examining the obese-asthma interplay, it is important to assess whether this association is mediated by sex, race, or ethnicity. Obesity seems to be a significant risk factor for developing asthma in women.[8,15,16] However, the role of obesity in men is less certain, with conflicting results. There are numerous studies reporting that obesity does not increase the risk of developing asthma in men.[3,16,17] In contrast, Beuther and Sutherland,[10] as well Huovinen and colleagues,[18] reported that the risk of developing asthma is similar in both women and men, although there was a trend toward greater risk in women. Gender in combination with race and ethnicity could explain the inconsistent data in men. In a CDC survey from the 2000 BRFSS the obesity-asthma association was found in men, but only in Hispanic and black people.[15]

The role of race and ethnicity in the relationship between obesity and asthma should be examined. Similar obesity-asthma associations have been shown in Chinese, Norwegian, and Indian populations.[19–22] Kim and Camargo[15] showed the obesity-asthma association in black and Hispanic people. In the 2009 to 2010 BRFSS, obesity was determined to be a risk factor in both white and black people.[23] The Black Women's Health Study followed more than 40,000 women over 10-year and found an increased incidence in asthma in the overweight and obese population, with a dose-response relationship.[24] These data suggest that the association between obesity and asthma exists in a diverse population.

The controversy surrounding obesity's effect on asthma in men versus women not only exists in the adult population but also in the pediatric population. Contrary to the adult studies, many pediatric studies show a greater association of obesity as a risk factor for boys instead of girls.[12,25] One study comparing lung function of boys and girls aged 6 to17 years found that obese boys had significantly worse airflow obstruction compared with their normal-weight counterparts, whereas in girls obesity did not cause any difference in level of airflow obstruction compared with the normal-weight asthmatics.[26]

In the pediatric population, a few studies have examined the role of race in the risk of asthma. One pediatric study found that, although obese Hispanic and white individuals had increases in incidence of asthma, the increase was significantly higher in Asian/Pacific Islanders and was attenuated in black individuals.[12]

PATHOPHYSIOLOGY
Obesity and Lung Function

An increase of BMI leads to airway changes independent of asthma. The most significant changes noted with increased BMIs occur in lung volumes. There are significant reductions in functional residual capacity (FRC) and expiratory reserve volume (ERV). In general, these changes only become evident when patients reach BMI greater than 30. At this level of obesity, the FRC and ERV are 75% and 45%, respectively, that of subjects with a BMI of 20. In addition, patients with BMI greater than 30 develop mild changes in total lung capacity, vital lung capacity, and residual volume.[27] With increased BMI, there can be proportional decreases in both the forced expiratory volume in 1 second (FEV$_1$) and forced vital capacity (FVC),[28] or more profound reduction in FVC,[29] resulting in a normal or increased FEV$_1$/FVC. However, because obese individuals breathe at lower lung volumes, the resulting airway narrowing may contribute to heightened airway reactivity.[30–33] **Table 2** presents a summary chart of lung function in obese asthmatics.

Obesity and Airway Inflammation

Obesity is a state of chronic low-grade inflammation with increased adipocyte-driven proinflammatory activity.[34,35] Adipocytes secrete hormones, including leptin and adiponectin. These adipokines are being investigated to determine their role in inflammatory states such as asthma. In addition, there is increased secretion of tumor necrosis factor alpha, interleukin-6, plasminogen activator factor-1, and nitric oxide, as well as increased infiltration of macrophages.[35,36] Adipokine secretion and macrophage infiltration creates systemic and local inflammation.

Several studies have determined that inflammation in obese asthmatics is not the traditional eosinophilic/T helper 2 (TH2) inflammation. This difference in the inflammatory response could explain the poor response to standard asthma therapy. Several studies have shown that increasing BMI is inversely related to sputum eosinophils, fraction of exhaled nitric oxide (F$_{ENO}$; a marker of eosinophilic inflammation), or both.[37–39] In contrast, there are also studies that did not find any significant relationship between body mass index and sputum eosinophils.[40]

Neutrophil-predominant inflammation is associated with difficult-to-control forms of asthma. Therefore, because obesity is associated with a more severe phenotype of asthma (discussed later), some obese asthmatics show a trend toward neutrophilic inflammation. Several studies have described a group of obese women with asthma who have neutrophil-predominant inflammation.[41,42] In addition, there is a decrease in airway neutrophils with weight loss by both dietary changes and by exercise.[43]

Table 2 Lung function in obese asthmatics (BMI>30)	
Lung Function	**Observed Effect**
FRC	Decreased
ERV	Decreased
Total lung capacity	Mildly reduced
Vital lung capacity	Mildly reduced
FEV$_1$/FVC	Normal/increased
Spirometry interpretation	Restrictive

CLINICAL FEATURES
What Are Phenotypes and Cluster Analyses?

Asthma is a heterogeneous disease. The additional comorbidity of obesity adds to the complexity by creating new obese-asthma phenotypes. Phenotypes are defined as the set of observable characteristics of an organism that are produced by the interactions of the genotype and the environment.[44] In asthma, phenotypes are based on several factors, including age of onset, smoke exposure, atopy, inflammatory infiltrates, severity of disease, and response to standard medications. With a better understanding of these phenotypes, clinicians can more effectively treat this population of patients.

Cluster analysis uses multivariate mathematical algorithms to quantify similarities between individuals within a population based on multiple specific variables, and then groups individuals into clusters based on their similarities.[45] By using cluster analyses, researchers are able to objectively define these phenotypes, including the newly described obese-asthma phenotypes (**Table 3**).

Obese Versus Lean Asthmatics: Differences in Presentation

Cluster analyses and clinical observation have shown that obese asthmatics are not a uniform group. Several cluster analyses have identified two major groups of obese asthmatics that are categorized by age of onset of asthma symptoms as well as TH2 inflammation. These groups are designated as early-onset and late-onset obese asthma. In comparisons of both groups of obese asthmatics with their lean counterparts, more of the obese/overweight individuals take controller medications. They also had more continuous respiratory symptoms and lower quality-of-life scores than their lean counterparts.[46–48] In the cluster analysis by Sutherland and colleagues,[72] both obese groups had similar lung impairment, levels of adipokines, markers of systemic inflammation, and immunoglobulin E (IgE), the last of which is a differentiating factor between the two phenotypes in other analyses (discussed later).

Early-onset Obesity Associated Asthma

The early-onset group has asthma symptoms before 12 years of age with obesity playing a complicating role. The early-onset asthma affects male and female patients equally and is atopic in nature, with members of this group having increased IgE levels. They also have severely decreased airway function, significant airway hyperresponsiveness, and poor asthma control. Airway inflammation is dominated by eosinophilic infiltration with high exhaled nitric oxide levels.[47]

Table 3	
Obese-asthma phenotypes (early onset vs late onset)	
Early-onset Asthma	**Late-onset Asthma**
Onset<12 y	Onset>12 y
Male = Female	Female > Male
Atopic	Nonatopic
Severe decrease in airway function (FEV$_1$, FVC)	Minimal airway obstruction (FEV$_1$, FVC)
Significant airway hyperresponsiveness	Less airway hyperresponsiveness
Higher symptom score	Lower symptoms score
Eosinophilic airway infiltration	Neutrophilic infiltration
High TH2 biomarkers	Low TH2 biomarkers

Late-onset Obesity Associated Asthma

In contrast, obese patients with late-onset asthma are predominantly female, presenting after 12 years of age, and lacking atopic characteristics. Pulmonary function testing shows minimal airway obstruction and less airway hyperresponsiveness, with better asthma control and lower symptom scores than the early-onset asthmatics. This phenotype has a TH2 low profile with predominant neutrophil infiltration, low IgE, and low eosinophilic infiltration.[49]

Clinical Outcomes

In comparisons of the clinical outcomes of obese asthmatics with their lean counterparts, the difference is apparent. The early-onset asthmatic population required more oral corticosteroid tapers, emergency department visits, hospital admissions, intensive care unit admissions, and mechanical ventilation. In addition, they had a higher incidence of pneumonia than lean asthmatics.[47] Obese asthmatics were more likely to be classified as severe asthmatics, miss more days of work, and report continuous symptoms.[13] In addition, obesity has a more detrimental effect on the lung function of children and adolescents compared with adults.[50]

OBESE ASTHMATICS AND STANDARD ASTHMA TREATMENT

Obese asthmatics' reduced response to standard therapy makes them a particularly challenging group of asthmatics to manage. This group of patients has a reduced response to the first-line therapy for persistent asthmatics, inhaled corticosteroids, which leads them to present with more difficult-to-control asthma. Peters-Golden and colleagues[51] showed that patients on beclomethasone with higher BMIs had less asthma control days (ACD), whereas the number of ACD did not decrease with increasing BMI in patients on montelukast. When treated with budesonide, the normal-weight group in another study had a more significant reduction in Feno as well as symptom improvement compared with the overweight group (BMI>25 kg/m^2). There was no significant difference in airway hyper-reactivity as examined by the methacholine provocation concentration (PC20) which reduces FEV1 by 20%.[52]

In a post-hoc analysis of data from multiple clinical trials, in both the obese and non-obese groups, fluticasone in combination with salmeterol provided better asthma control than fluticasone alone in more than 1200 patients with moderate asthma. The obese group continued to have poorer asthma control with these controllers compared with the normal-weight group.[53] In comparisons of inhaled corticosteroid (ICS), ICS/short acting beta agonist (SABA), and montelukast, ICS and ICS/SABA were more effective in asthma treatment than montelukast.[54] The effectiveness of low dose theophylline as add-on treatment in asthma (LODO) trial, with a cohort of 488 women, of whom 47% were obese, examined differences in presentation and response to add-on treatment with placebo, montelukast, or theophylline. With add-on theophylline, obese asthmatics had a trend toward more frequent asthma exacerbations compared with lean asthmatics. There was no difference with montelukast treatment.[55] None of the studies examining the response to controller medications among obese asthmatics has stratified them into the two phenotypes: early versus late onset of asthma.

TREATMENT OPTIONS FOR OBESE ASTHMATICS
Weight Loss

Because of the limited effectiveness of standard forms of medical therapy, new avenues for managing obese asthmatics must be explored. If obesity is a contributing risk factor for not only development but also severity of disease, then weight reduction is an obvious approach to preventing and treating asthma in this population. Weight is one of the only modifiable risk factors for asthma. There are multiple studies of value of dietary and surgical weight loss for improved asthma outcomes.[56-64] The results have been mixed but encouraging and are reviewed in detail elsewhere in this issue.

Role of Diet in Asthma Development and Control

In obese asthmatics, the specific contents of the diet, including fats, sugar, and low nutrients, may contribute to the chronic inflammatory state. Even a single high-fat meal has an immediate effect on inflammatory cells as well lung function. In one study, patients were given 1 high-fat meal and were monitored for 4 hours. There was a significant decrease in the response to bronchodilators as well as a rapid decrease in FEV_1/FVC ratio after the high-fat meal. In addition, sputum showed an increase in airway neutrophils.[65] This finding is consistent with previously discussed studies that found a neutrophil-predominant inflammation in obese asthmatics.

There have been several studies of the use of dietary supplementation or alteration as a means to develop better asthma control. Cochrane Reviews examining the role of supplementation with vitamin C, selenium, and low-salt diets have shown no promising evidence for benefits on asthma symptoms.[66-68] Vitamin C may have some indication for exercise-induced asthma, but its use must be assessed further.[68] At present, there is a clinical trial (Dietary Approaches to Stop Hypertension [DASH]) of the efficacy of diet as an adjunct therapy to standard adult therapy in uncontrolled asthmatics. The DASH diet encompasses fresh fruit, vegetables, nuts, and antioxidant nutrients (vitamins A, C, E; and zinc).[69] In addition, vitamin D has been hypothesized to play a role in the interplay between obesity and asthma. Vitamin D levels are inversely correlated with BMI and with asthma severity,[70-72] and higher serum levels are associated with improved in vitro sensitivity to glucocorticoids.[72]

The Mediterranean diet has also proved in many studies to have protective effects on both asthma and allergic rhinitis.[73-76] One cross-sectional study examined 174 adults with asthma and defined the patients as controlled and uncontrolled asthmatics using FEV_1, Fe_{NO}, and asthma control questionnaire (ACQ). Diet was analyzed using the alternate Mediterranean Diet Score (aMED). Controlled asthmatics had a higher aMED score, greater intake of fresh fruit, and lower ethanol intake compared with the uncontrolled asthmatics. Asthmatics who adhered to a Mediterranean diet had a 78% reduced risk of having uncontrolled asthma.[75] However, the role of diet and nutrition in development of asthma remains controversial and is reviewed in greater detail elsewhere in this issue.

Old Medications, New Use

With the complicated nature of the obese-asthma phenotypes and resistance to standard asthma therapy, new treatments must be evaluated. Statins, which are prescribed for hyperlipidemia, have been found to have antiinflammatory effects, prevent remodeling of lung tissue, and improve lung function.[77-79] There have been varying results of the efficacy of statins in asthma, but the key may be in the selection of the patient population that will benefit from this form of treatment. A recent study hypothesized that it was the severe asthmatics, most of whom were obese, that would benefit from statins as an add-on therapy. This retrospective study examined 165 adult patients, who were divided into 2 groups: those on statins (who were mostly female and obese) and those not on statins. Their charts were examined for asthma control test (ACT) scores as a primary measure of asthma control.

Patients who were on statins had significantly increased ACT scores compared with their counterparts. This finding remained true even when comorbidities like gastro-esophageal reflux disease (GERD), obstructive sleep apnea (OSA), and smoking were accounted for.[80]

COMORBID CONFOUNDERS IN OBESE ASTHMATICS

It is difficult to isolate obesity and asthma from other associated comorbidities that are common in obese patients, such as GERD, OSA, and depression.[39,81] GERD was pre-viously thought to be a contributor to asthma symptoms, but in several studies, including a Cochrane Review, GERD treatment did not produce improvement in asthma symptoms.[82,83] In obese asthmatics, it may be OSA but not GERD that con-tributes significantly to poor asthma control.[84] OSA[84,85] and depression[86,87] are known to contribute to poorly controlled asthma. Obese individuals with depression or anxiety have the highest risk (odds ratio, 2.93) of incident asthma compared with other groups in a prospective study of more than 20,000 adults.[88] Although these con-ditions may be associated with asthma-like symptoms, their presence does not fully explain the creation of this obese-asthma phenotype. Instead, these comorbidities may contribute to additional barriers in the complete management of symptoms. Because of the complexity of the conditions involved, obesity-associated asthma is a multifaceted condition requiring a multidisciplinary approach when developing a treatment plan (**Fig. 1**).

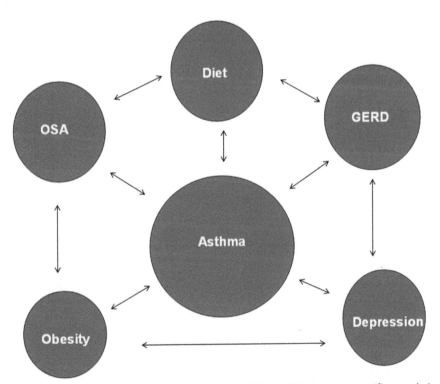

Fig. 1. The interplay between asthma and its comorbid conditions plays a significant role in the management of the obese asthmatic patient.

SUMMARY/FUTURE CONSIDERATIONS

The increasing incidence of obesity and asthma has led to the development of 2 newly defined obese-asthma phenotypes, each characterized by the age of onset of asthma. Both groups of obese asthmatics have symptoms that are more difficult to control than those of lean asthmatics. Members of the late-onset group are more likely to be nonatopic. In order to provide better treatment of these patients, physicians must be able to recognize the barriers involved in managing their asthma. These issues include, most significantly, resistance to inhaled corticosteroids as well as the additional complexity of comorbid conditions. Treatment plans need to be multidisciplinary, including asthma therapy, weight management, dietary changes, and mental health care.

With the help of cluster analyses clinicians are just beginning to make progress in understanding obese asthmatics. More knowledge about what characterizes these phenotypes, as well as an in-depth understanding of the underlying pathophysiology, or endotype, will allow more effective and personalized forms of asthma treatments to be developed. At present, there are investigations examining the role of adiponectin and leptin in the pathogenesis of this phenotype. In the future, there may be treatments to modulate adipokine levels or activity in order to obtain better asthma control. Investigators should assess how another comorbidity of obesity, diabetes, may affect the severity of asthma and prospectively examine the protective, antiinflammatory potential of some common diabetes and cardiac medications in refractory asthmatics. Furthermore, an interesting subpopulation to study would be the elderly, in whom many of these comorbidities converge. Futures studies focusing on obese asthmatics should differentiate the two distinct phenotypes, early-onset versus late-onset asthma, associated with obesity, while studying the underlying pathophysiology and determining the effectiveness of alternative treatments.

REFERENCES

1. Ma J, Xiao L. Association of general and central obesity and atopic and nonatopic asthma in US adults. J Asthma 2013;50(4):395–402.
2. Tavasoli S, Eghtesadi S, Heidarnazhad H, et al. Central obesity and asthma outcomes in adults diagnosed with asthma. J Asthma 2013;50(2):180–7.
3. Kronander UN, Falkenberg M, Zetterstrom O. Prevalence and incidence of asthma related to waist circumference and BMI in a Swedish community sample. Respir Med 2004;98(11):1108–16.
4. WHO. Obesity and overweight. [cited 2014]. Available at: http://www.who.int/mediacentre/factsheets/fs311/en/#.
5. Ogden CL, Carroll MD, Kit BK, et al. Prevalence of obesity in the United States, 2009–2010. NCHS data brief, No. 82. Hyattsville (MD): National Center for Health Statistics; 2012.
6. CDC. Behavioral risk factor surveillance system: obesity trends among U.S. adults. 2011. Available at: www.cdc.gov/brfss.
7. CDC. Asthma in the US. Vital signs. 2011. Available at: www.cdc.gov/vitalsigns/asthma.
8. Camargo C, Weiss S, Zhang S, et al. Prospective study of body mass index, weight change, and risk of adult-onset asthma in women. Arch Intern Med 1999;159(21):2582–8.
9. Rodríguez M, Winkleby M, Ahn D, et al. Identification of population subgroups of children and adolescents with high asthma prevalence: findings from the third

National Health and Nutrition Examination Survey. Arch Pediatr Adolesc Med 2002;156(3):269–75.

10. Beuther DA, Sutherland ER. Overweight, obesity, and incident asthma - a meta-analysis of prospective epidemiologic studies. Am J Respir Crit Care Med 2007; 175(7):661–6.

11. Brüske I, Flexeder C, Heinrich J. Body mass index and the incidence of asthma in children. Curr Opin Allergy Clin Immunol 2014;14(2):155–60.

12. Black MH, Zhou H, Takayanagi M, et al. Increased asthma risk and asthma-related health care complications associated with childhood obesity. Am J Epidemiol 2013;178(7):1120–8.

13. Taylor B, Mannino D, Brown C, et al. Body mass index and asthma severity in the National Asthma Survey. Thorax 2008;63(1):14–20.

14. Black MH, Smith N, Porter AH, et al. Higher prevalence of obesity among children with asthma. Obesity (Silver Spring) 2012;20(5):1041–7.

15. Kim S, Camargo CA. Sex-race differences in the relationship between obesity and asthma: the behavioral risk factor surveillance system, 2000. Ann Epidemiol 2003;13(10):666–73.

16. Hancox RJ, Milne BJ, Poulton R, et al. Sex differences in the relation between body mass index and asthma and atopy in a birth cohort. Am J Respir Crit Care Med 2005;171(5):440–5.

17. Beckett WS, Jacobs DR, Yu X, et al. Asthma is associated with weight gain in females but not males, independent of physical activity. Am J Respir Crit Care Med 2001;164(11):2045–50.

18. Huovinen E, Kaprio J, Koskenvuo M. Factors associated to lifestyle and risk of adult onset asthma. Respir Med 2003;97(3):273–80.

19. Wang D, Qian Z, Wang J, et al. Gender-specific differences in associations of overweight and obesity with asthma and asthma-related symptoms in 30,056 children: result from 25 districts of northeastern China. J Asthma 2014;51(5): 508–14.

20. Willeboordse M, et al. Sex differences in the relationship between asthma and overweight in Dutch children: a survey study. PLoS One 2013;8(10):e77574.

21. Nystad W, Meyer HE, Nafstad P, et al. Body mass index in relation to adult asthma among 135,000 Norwegian men and women. Am J Epidemiol 2004; 160(10):969–76.

22. Mishra V. Effect of obesity on asthma among adult Indian women. Int J Obes Relat Metab Disord 2004;28(8):1048–58.

23. Zahran H, Bailey C. Factors associated with asthma prevalence among racial and ethnic groups–United States, 2009-2010 behavioral risk factor surveillance system. J Asthma 2013;50(6):583–9.

24. Coogan PF, Palmer JR, O'Connor GT, et al. Body mass index and asthma incidence in the Black Women's Health Study. J Allergy Clin Immunol 2009;123(1): 89–95.

25. Borrell LN, Nguyen EA, Roth LA, et al. Childhood obesity and asthma control in the GALA II and SAGE II Studies. Am J Respir Crit Care Med 2013;187(7): 697–702.

26. Lang JE, Holbrook JT, Wise RA, et al. Obesity in children with poorly controlled asthma: sex differences. Pediatr Pulmonol 2013;48(9):847–56.

27. Jones R, Nzekwu M. The effects of body mass index on lung volumes. Chest 2006;130(3):827–33.

28. Collins L, Hoberty P, Walker J, et al. The effect of body fat distribution on pulmonary function tests. Chest 1995;107:1298–302.

29. Lazarus R, Sparrow D, Weiss S. Effect of obesity and fat distribution on ventilatory function. Chest 1997;111:891–8.
30. Chinn S, Jarvis D, Burney P. Relation of bronchial responsiveness to body mass index in the ECRHS. Thorax 2002;57(12):1028–33.
31. Litonjua A, Sparrow D, Celedon J, et al. Association of body mass index with the development of methacholine airway hyperresponsiveness in men: the Normative Aging Study. Thorax 2002;57(7):581–5.
32. Sposato B, Scalese M, Scichilone N. BMI can influence adult males' and females' airway hyperresponsiveness differently. Multidiscip Respir Med 2012; 7(1):45.
33. Sharma S, Tailor A, Warrington R, et al. Is obesity associated with an increased risk for airway hyperresponsiveness and development of asthma? Allergy Asthma Clin Immunol 2008;4(2):51–8.
34. Shore SA. Obesity and asthma: possible mechanisms. J Allergy Clin Immunol 2008;121(5):1087–93.
35. Wellen K, Hotamisligil G. Inflammation, stress, and diabetes. J Clin Invest 2005; 115(5):1111–9.
36. Weisberg SP, McCann D, Desai M, et al. Obesity is associated with macrophage accumulation in adipose tissue. J Clin Invest 2003;112(12):1796–808.
37. Quinto KB, Zuraw BL, Poon KYT, et al. The association of obesity and asthma severity and control in children. J Allergy Clin Immunol 2011;128(5):964–9.
38. Komakula S, Khatri S, Mermis J, et al. Body mass index is associated with reduced exhaled nitric oxide and higher exhaled 8-isoprostanes in asthmatics. Respir Res 2007;8(1):32.
39. Van Veen IH, Ten Brinke A, Sterk PJ, et al. Airway inflammation in obese and nonobese patients with difficult-to-treat asthma. Allergy 2008;63(5):570–4.
40. Todd DC, Armstrong S, D'Silva L, et al. Effect of obesity on airway inflammation: a cross-sectional analysis of body mass index and sputum cell counts. Clin Exp Allergy 2007;37(7):1049–54.
41. Scott HA, Gibson PG, Garg ML, et al. Airway inflammation is augmented by obesity and fatty acids in asthma. Eur Respir J 2011;38(3):594–602.
42. Telenga ED, Tideman SW, Kerstjens HAM, et al. Obesity in asthma: more neutrophilic inflammation as a possible explanation for a reduced treatment response. Allergy 2012;67(8):1060–8.
43. Scott HA, Gibson PG, Garg ML, et al. Dietary restriction and exercise improve airway inflammation and clinical outcomes in overweight and obese asthma: a randomized trial. Clin Exp Allergy 2013;43(1):36–49.
44. Merriam-Webster, n.d.W. Merriam-Webster.com. 2014. [cited February 6, 2014]. Available at: http://www.merriam-webster.com/dictionary/phenotype.
45. Everitt B, Landau S, Leese M. Cluster analysis. 4th edition. London: Arnold; 2001.
46. Haldar P, Pavord ID, Shaw DE, et al. Cluster analysis and clinical asthma phenotypes. Am J Respir Crit Care Med 2008;178:218–24.
47. Holguin F, Bleecker ER, Busse WW, et al. Obesity and asthma: an association modified by age of asthma onset. J Allergy Clin Immunol 2011;127(6): 1486–93.e2.
48. Moore WC, Meyers DA, Wenzel SE, et al. Identification of asthma phenotypes using cluster analysis in the severe asthma research program. Am J Respir Crit Care Med 2010;181:315–23.
49. Rasmussen F, Hancox RJ. Mechanisms of obesity in asthma. Curr Opin Allergy Clin Immunol 2014;14(1):35–43.

50. Lang JE, Hossain J, Dixon AE, et al. Does age impact the obese asthma phenotype?: longitudinal asthma control, airway function, and airflow perception among mild persistent asthmatics. Chest 2011;140(6):1524–33.
51. Peters-Golden M, Swern A, Bird SS, et al. Influence of body mass index on the response to asthma controller agents. Eur Respir J 2006;27(3):495–503.
52. Anderson WJ, Lipworth BJ. Does body mass index influence responsiveness to inhaled corticosteroids in persistent asthma? Ann Allergy Asthma Immunol 2012;108(4):237–42.
53. Boulet LP, Franssen E. Influence of obesity on response to fluticasone with or without salmeterol in moderate asthma. Respir Med 2007;101(11):2240–7.
54. Camargo CA Jr, Boulet LP, Sutherland ER, et al. Body mass index and response to asthma therapy: fluticasone propionate/salmeterol versus montelukast. J Asthma 2010;47(1):76–82.
55. Dixon AE, Shade DM, Cohen RI, et al. Effect of obesity on clinical presentation and response to treatment in asthma. J Asthma 2006;43(7):553–8.
56. Stenius-Aarniala B, et al. Immediate and long term effects of weight reduction in obese people with asthma: randomised controlled study. BMJ 2000;320(7238): 827–32.
57. Johnson JB, Summer W, Cutler RG, et al. Alternate day calorie restriction improves clinical findings and reduces markers of oxidative stress and inflammation in overweight adults with moderate asthma. Free Radic Biol Med 2007; 42(5):665–74.
58. Simard B, Turcotte H, Marceau P, et al. Asthma and sleep apnea in patients with morbid obesity: outcome after bariatric surgery. Obes Surg 2004;14(10): 1381–8.
59. Maniscalco M, Zedda A, Faraone S, et al. Weight loss and asthma control in severely obese asthmatic females. Respir Med 2008;102(1):102–8.
60. Lombardi C, Gargioni S, Gardinazzi A, et al. Impact of bariatric surgery on pulmonary function and nitric oxide in asthmatic and non-asthmatic obese patients. J Asthma 2011;48(6):553–7.
61. Reddy R, Baptist A, Fan Z, et al. The effects of bariatric surgery on asthma severity. Obes Surg 2011;21(2):200–6.
62. Hewitt S, Humerfelt S, Søvik T, et al. Long-term improvements in pulmonary function 5 years after bariatric surgery. Obes Surg 2014;24(5):705–11. http://dx.doi.org/10.1007/s11695-013-1159-9.
63. Dixon AE, Pratley RE, Forgione PM, et al. Effects of obesity and bariatric surgery on airway hyperresponsiveness, asthma control, and inflammation. J Allergy Clin Immunol 2011;128(3):508–15.e2.
64. Adeniyi FB, Young T. Weight loss interventions for chronic asthma. Cochrane Database Syst Rev 2012;(7):CD009339.
65. Wood LG, Garg ML, Gibson PG. A high-fat challenge increases airway inflammation and impairs bronchodilator recovery in asthma. J Allergy Clin Immunol 2011;127(5):1133–40.
66. Allam MF, Lucane RA. Selenium supplementation for asthma. Cochrane Database Syst Rev 2004;(2):CD003538.
67. Pogson Z, McKeever T. Dietary sodium manipulation and asthma. Cochrane Database Syst Rev 2011;(3):CD000436.
68. Milan S, Hart A, Wilkinson M. Vitamin C for asthma and exercise-induced bronchoconstriction. Cochrane Database Syst Rev 2013;(10):CD010391.
69. Ma J, Strub P, Lavori PW, et al. DASH for asthma: a pilot study of the DASH diet in not-well-controlled adult asthma. Contemp Clin Trials 2013;35(2):55–67.

70. Paul G, Brehm J, Alcorn J, et al. Vitamin D and asthma. Am J Respir Crit Care Med 2012;185(2):124–32.
71. Korn S, Hubner M, Jung M, et al. Severe and uncontrolled adult asthma is associated with vitamin D insufficiency and deficiency. Respir Res 2013;14(1):25.
72. Sutherland E, Goleva E, Jackson L, et al. Vitamin D levels, lung function and steroid response in adult asthma. Am J Respir Crit Care Med 2010;181:699–704.
73. Chatzi L, Apostolaki G, Bibakis I, et al. Protective effect of fruits, vegetables and the Mediterranean diet on asthma and allergies among children in Crete. Thorax 2007;62(8):677–83.
74. Garcia-Marcos L, Canflanca IM, Garrido JB, et al. Relationship of asthma and rhinoconjunctivitis with obesity, exercise and Mediterranean diet in Spanish schoolchildren. Thorax 2007;62(6):503–8.
75. Barros R, Moreira A, Fonseca J, et al. Adherence to the Mediterranean diet and fresh fruit intake are associated with improved asthma control. Allergy 2008; 63(7):917–23.
76. De Batlle J, Garcia-Aymerich J, Barraza-Villarreal A, et al. Mediterranean diet is associated with reduced asthma and rhinitis in Mexican children. Allergy 2008; 63(10):1310–6.
77. McKay A, Leung BP, McInnes IB, et al. A novel anti-inflammatory role of simvastatin in a murine model of allergic asthma. J Immunol 2004;172(5):2903–8.
78. Zeki AA, Bratt JM, Rabowsky M, et al. Simvastatin inhibits goblet cell hyperplasia and lung arginase in a mouse model of allergic asthma: a novel treatment for airway remodeling? Transl Res 2010;156(6):335–49.
79. Huang CC, Chan WL, Chen YC, et al. Statin use in patients with asthma: a nationwide population-based study. Eur J Clin Invest 2011;41(5):507–12.
80. Zeki AA, Oldham J, Wilson M. Statin use and asthma control in patients with severe asthma. BMJ Open 2013;3(8). pii:e003314.
81. Bhattacharya R, Shen C, Sambamoorthi U. Excess risk of chronic physical conditions associated with depression and anxiety. BMC Psychiatry 2014;14:10.
82. Gibson P, Henry R, Coughlan J. Gastro-oesophageal reflux treatment for asthma in adults and children. Cochrane Database Syst Rev 2003;(2):CD001496.
83. McCallister JW, Parsons JP, Mastronarde JG. The relationship between gastroesophageal reflux and asthma: an update. Ther Adv Respir Dis 2011;5(2): 143–50.
84. Dixon AE, Clerisme-Beaty EM, Sugar EA, et al. Effects of obstructive sleep apnea and gastroesophageal reflux disease on asthma control in obesity. J Asthma 2011;48(7):707–13.
85. Verhulst SL, Aerts L, Jacobs S, et al. Sleep-disordered breathing, obesity, and airway inflammation in children and adolescents. Chest 2008;134(6):1169–75.
86. Yonas M, Marsland A, Emeremni C, et al. Depressive symptomatology, quality of life and disease control among individuals with well-characterized severe asthma. J Asthma 2013;50(8):884–90.
87. Krauskopf K, Sofianou A, Goel M, et al. Depressive symptoms, low adherence, and poor asthma outcomes in the elderly. J Asthma 2013;50(3):260–6.
88. Brumpton B, Leivseth L, Romundstad P, et al. The joint association of anxiety, depression and obesity with incident asthma in adults: the HUNT study. Int J Epidemiol 2013;42(5):1455–63.

Childhood Obesity and Risk of Allergy or Asthma

Dinesh Raj, MD[a], Sushil K. Kabra, MD[b], Rakesh Lodha, MD[b],*

KEYWORDS

- Obesity • Asthma • Allergy • Airway inflammation • Adipokines

KEY POINTS

- There has been a simultaneous increase in the prevalence of obesity and allergic disorders in children, suggesting a possible link between the two.
- Obesity is associated more often with nonatopic asthma than atopic asthma, suggesting noneosinophilic inflammation and Th1 polarization.
- The evidence for the role of obesity in the augmentation of other allergic disorders is conflicting.
- The mechanisms of obesity-associated asthma possibly include deranged lung function, systemic/airway inflammation influenced by adipokines, comorbidities, and shared factors (diet, sedentary lifestyle, and genetics).

INTRODUCTION

Allergic diseases are the most common chronic diseases in children around the world. The prevalence of allergic diseases especially asthma has been found to be increasing over last 2 decades.[1,2] The prevalence of obesity has also increased tremendously over last 3 decades.[3] A simultaneous increment in the prevalence of both obesity and asthma/allergic diseases suggests a possible link between the two. Despite data suggesting the epidemiologic link between asthma and obesity, the relationship remains unclear and many confounders (gender, ethnicity, genetic factors, and comorbidities) are likely to influence the obesity–asthma link.

The aim of the current review was to focus on the consequences of obesity on allergic diseases, especially asthma in children and adolescents, and to evaluate the available evidence on the possible mechanisms.

EPIDEMIOLOGY OF OBESITY AND ALLERGIC DISEASES IN CHILDREN

In the National Health and Nutrition Examination Survey (NHANES) for 2009 through 2010, the prevalence of obesity was 16.9% in US children and adolescents (18.6%

The authors have nothing to disclose.
[a] Department of Pediatrics, Holy Family Hospital, Okhla, New Delhi 110025, India; [b] Department of Pediatrics, All India Institute of Medical Sciences, Ansari Nagar, New Delhi 110029, India
* Corresponding author.
E-mail address: rakesh_lodha@hotmail.com

Immunol Allergy Clin N Am 34 (2014) 753–765
http://dx.doi.org/10.1016/j.iac.2014.07.001
0889-8561/14/$ – see front matter © 2014 Elsevier Inc. All rights reserved.

in boys and 15.0% in girls).[3] Since 1980, the prevalence of obesity in children and adolescents has tripled. Asthma prevalence in children and adolescents (0–17 years) has increased from 3.6% in 1980% to 9.5% in 2008 through 2010.[1] The prevalence of allergic diseases (food and skin allergies) has similarly increased from 1997 to 2011 in children younger than 18 years in the United States.[2] Both asthma and obesity are more prevalent in children from low socioeconomic strata and minority populations.[1,3]

Prospective, population-based studies have shown an increased risk of incident asthma in children and adults with a greater body mass index (BMI).[4–8] Gender-based differences have been observed in some studies, with a stronger association between BMI and asthma among girls compared with boys.[4,9–11] Reports from the International Study of Asthma and Allergies in Childhood (ISAAC) Phase Three study involving 6- and 7-year-olds from 17 countries, and 13- and 14-year-olds from 35 countries, have shown significant association between overweight/obesity and asthma/eczema symptoms, but not with rhinoconjunctivitis.[12] Data from developing countries are still lacking on the association between obesity and asthma in children. We have been following a pediatric asthmatic cohort over last 5 years; the mean BMI of 240 children in this cohort was 15.3 ± 2.6 kg/m^2, with only 2% overweight and obese individuals.

A recent population based longitudinal study assessing health records of 623,358 patients aged 6 to 19 years suggested that obese individuals are not only at risk of asthma, but also more likely to have severe asthma, resulting in greater health care utilization, asthma exacerbations, and aggressive asthma treatment.[13]

OBESITY AND RISK OF ATOPY/ALLERGY

Evidence is conflicting on the potential role of obesity on the development of allergy or atopy in childhood. The data from the NHANES III (1988–1994) showed significant association between BMI and asthma, but no association between BMI and atopy (as defined by positive skin prick testing) after adjusting for confounders.[14] Subsequent reports from the NHANES for 1998 through 2006 survey found a stronger association between obesity and current asthma in nonatopic children (odds ratio [OR], 2.46; 95% CI, 1.21–5.02) than atopic children (OR, 1.34; 95% CI, 0.70–2.57).[15] A large, multicenter, cross-sectional study of adults (aged 20–44 years) did not find any association between raised BMI and atopy (sensitization to dust mite, cat, grass, specific immunoglobulin [Ig]E against these allergens, and total IgE).[16]

Similarly, a large, multicenter, cross-sectional study from 8 Spanish cities concluded that obese schoolchildren (6- and 7-year-olds) were at a greater risk of nonallergic asthma than nonobese subjects, whereas the risk of allergic asthma was similar.[17] This was a questionnaire-based study and the authors used rhinoconjunctivitis as a marker of atopy. A study of Portuguese schoolchildren found increased prevalence of overweight/obesity in atopic children compared with nonatopic children.[18]

Gender has also been found to affect the relationship between obesity and atopy. Collective data from Caucasian Australian children suggested that higher BMI was associated with an higher prevalence of atopy in girls only.[19] A somewhat similar observation has been made in a birth cohort study from New Zealand.[20] The cohort was evaluated at various occasions between age 9 and 26 years. A higher BMI was associated with asthma and atopy in women only. BMI has also been associated with increased prevalence of atopy and allergic symptoms in Taiwanese adolescent girls.[21]

As evident from these studies, there is no consistent evidence of association between obesity and atopy. The obesity–asthma relationship is also stronger in nonatopic asthma compared with atopic asthma, with possible effect modification by gender. The association of obesity with markers of allergic inflammation, like peripheral eosinophil counts and exhaled nitric oxide, is also not consistent. The studies are also heterogeneous in terms of definition of allergy or atopy, using self-reported allergic symptoms, parental questionnaires, skin prick testing, specific IgE levels, or total IgE levels.

The association between allergic diseases other than asthma and obesity is conflicting and not as consistent as the obesity–asthma link. A study in Japanese school children based on ISAAC questionnaires reported a positive relationship between obesity and asthma prevalence, and allergic dermatitis severity, but negative associations between obesity and allergic rhinitis and allergic conjunctivitis.[22] A large, retrospective, case control study in US children and adolescents with atopic dermatitis found a positive relation between obesity and atopic dermatitis (OR, 2.0; 95% CI, 1.22–3.26; P = .006).[23] The association was present when obesity started before 2 years of age but absent beyond 5 years of age. Differently, a study of Belgian schoolchildren found no relation between BMI and allergic symptoms (respiratory, eczema, and rhinoconjunctivitis).[24]

To summarize, the association between BMI and allergic disorders other than asthma is conflicting and is possibly modified by age, gender, ethnicity, and type of disease. The association between BMI and eczema is fairly consistent. However, there is no/inverse relationship between BMI and allergic rhinitis/rhinoconjunctivitis.

Table 1 summarizes the results of various studies evaluating the relation between obesity and allergic disorders.

IS OBESITY A CAUSE OR EFFECT OF ASTHMA: CAUSALITY AND REVERSE CAUSALITY?

The hypothesis of asthma preceding obesity is supported by the evidence that asthmatics receive frequent steroid bursts, are likely to exercise less fearing asthma symptoms, stay more indoors leading to increased exposure to indoor air pollution, and pursue a sedentary lifestyle. A prospective community based cross-sectional study of young adults followed up between 20 and 40 years found an association between asthma and obesity.[33] However, longitudinal follow-up of the cohort revealed that asthma preceded weight gain and subsequent obesity. Obesity was not associated with subsequent asthma. Childhood depressive symptoms possibly contributed to a major part of the asthma–obesity relation in this study. The authors stressed the role played by psychological factors during childhood, which may influence the obesity–asthma relationship in adolescence and adults. Further, there are data using Granger causality tests relating past asthma diagnosis with subsequent obesity.[34]

The evidence evaluating the obesity–asthma link in children has to be viewed carefully, because there are plaguing issues pertaining to definitions of asthma and obesity. Most of the studies have defined asthma using self- or parent-reported symptoms or physician-diagnosed asthma. Few studies have used stringent asthma diagnosis, including bronchodilation or bronchoprovocation tests. Similarly, obesity has been variously defined. Although most studies use BMI as a marker for adiposity using the World Health Organization definition of BMI as greater than 30 kg/m^2 or greater than the 95th percentile, other studies have used weight, weight for height z-score, waist circumference, conicity index, percent body fat, and skin fold thickness. The lack of uniformity in the definition of asthma and obesity is likely to affect the interpretation of the results and adds to the heterogeneity of evidence.

Table 1
Summary of studies evaluating the relation between obesity and allergy

Author,[Ref] Year Country	Studied	Sample Size/Study Population	Definition of Atopy	Summary of Findings
Fenger et al,[25] 2012 Denmark	Association between different adiposity measures and asthma/atopy/lung function	Population based study 3471 persons, 19–72 y	Specific IgE	All measures of adiposity associated with asthma (stronger in nonatopics than atopics)
Cibella et al,[26] 2011 Italy	Association between BMI and FENO/allergic sensitization	Cross-sectional epidemiologic study 708 children (10–16 y)	Skin prick tests, FENO	BMI not associated with high FENO, but independently related to asthma/allergic sensitization
Silverberg et al,[23] 2011 US	Association between obesity and atopic dermatitis	Retrospective, case-control study: 414 persons (1–21 y) with atopic dermatitis 828 healthy controls	Atopic dermatitis based on diagnostic criteria	Obesity was associated with increased risk and severity of atopic dermatitis
Visness et al,[15] 2010 US	Association between obesity and asthma in atopic and non atopic individuals	NHANES (2005–2006) 3387 individuals (1–19 y)	Specific IgE	Association stronger in nonatopics than atopics
Musaad et al,[27] 2009 US	Association of measures of obesity with allergic asthma	Cross-sectional case control study 1123 children (5–18 y)	Skin prick tests	Negative association between obesity and allergic sensitization among asthmatics
Spathopoulos et al,[28] 2009 Greece	Association of obesity with asthma/atopy	Cross-sectional study 2715 children (6–11 y)	Questionnaire based	High BMI independent risk factor for asthma/atopy
Chen et al,[29] 2009 Canada	Association between obesity and asthma in atopic and nonatopic individuals	Cross-sectional study 1997 adults (18–79 y)	Skin prick tests	Association between obesity and asthma stronger in nonatopics
Gysel et al,[24] 2009 Belgium	Association between BMI categories and atopy	Cross-sectional study 1576 children (3.4–14.8 y)	Skin prick tests	No difference in sensitization between normal weight and obese/overweight

Study	Objective	Design/Population	Measurement	Findings
Leung et al,[30] 2009 China	Association between adiposity markers and asthma/atopy	Cross-sectional study 486 school children	Specific IgE	No association between obesity and asthma/atopy
Ross et al,[31] 2009 US	Evaluation of the risk factors and comorbidities in children with asthma and obesity	Cross-sectional study 116 children (4–18 y)	Skin prick tests or specific IgE	No difference in proportion of atopy in obese and nonobese individuals
Garcia-Marcos et al,[17] 2008 Spain	Effect modification of allergy on asthma obesity relationship	Cross-sectional study 17,145 school children (6–7 y)	Presence of rhinoconjunctivitis based on questionnaires	Obese children at increased risk of nonallergic asthma than nonobese children
Silva et al,[18] 2007 Portugal	Association between BMI and atopic disease	Cross-sectional study 112 with atopy, 116 without atopy (5–16 y)	ISAAC questionnaire based diagnosis of asthma, AR, allergic eczema	Overweight/obesity more prevalent in atopic children
Hancox et al,[20] 2005 New Zealand	Relationship between BMI, asthma, and atopy	Prospective birth cohort of 1037 children followed for ≤26 y	Skin prick tests	Increased BMI associated with asthma and atopy in females only
Tantisira et al,[32] 2003 US	Relationship of BMI with measures of asthma severity	Baseline data of CAMP study (an RCT) 1041 children (5–12 y)	IgE and eosinophil counts	No association of atopy with BMI
Jarvis et al,[16] 2002 16 countries	Association between BMI and respiratory symptoms/atopy	ECRHS 13,909 adults (20–44 y)	Specific and total IgE	No association between BMI and atopy
von Mutius et al[14] 2001 US	Association of BMI with asthma/atopy	NHANES III (1988–1994), 7505 children (4–17 y)	Skin prick tests	After adjustment for confounders only asthma, not atopy, related to BMI

Abbreviations: AR, Allergic rhinitis; BMI, body mass index; CAMP, Childhood Asthma Management Program; ECRHS, European Community Respiratory Health Survey; FENO, fractional exhaled nitric oxide; Ig, immunoglobulin; ISAAC, International Study on Asthma and Allergy in Childhood; NHANES, National Health and Nutrition Examination Survey; RCT, randomized, controlled trial.

With many prospective studies from different countries, it has been observed that obesity is likely to precede asthma in most scenarios. However, there remains a likelihood of a subgroup of children (especially the early onset phenotype) in which asthma might precede obesity.

POSSIBLE MECHANISMS OF ASTHMA IN THE OBESE CHILDREN

The obesity–asthma link is complex and likely to be affected by many confounders. Obesity affects the lungs in multiple ways. These include changes in lung mechanics, augmentation of airway inflammation, common genetic basis, inflammatory effects of adipokines and cytokines, increased airway hyperresponsiveness, decreased physical activity, and effects of obesity related comorbidities (gastroesophageal reflux disease [GERD], sleep-disordered breathing [SDB]; **Box 1**).[35–37]

ADIPOKINES AND SYSTEMIC INFLAMMATION IN OBESITY: DO THESE AGGRAVATE OR CAUSE ASTHMA?

The adipose tissue in the obese is involved in the release of certain hormones (leptin, adiponectin, and resistin)[38] and cytokines (tumor necrosis factor-α, interleukin [IL]-6). These hormones and cytokines might be responsible for insulin resistance, hypertension, cardiovascular morbidities, metabolic disorders, and asthma related to obesity. Whether these adipokines and cytokines are involved in modifying the risk of asthma in obese children remains unclear.

Box 1
Proposed mechanisms responsible for obesity–asthma link

1. Inflammation
   - Adipokines (leptin, adiponectin, resistin, C-reactive protein, tumor necrosis factor-α, intereukin-6)
   - Airway inflammation
   - Oxidative stress
2. Lung mechanics
   - Reduced lung volumes
   - Poor lung function
   - Airway closure
3. Comorbidities
   - Gastroesophageal reflux disease
   - Sleep-disordered breathing
   - Dyslipidemia
4. Physical deconditioning/increased perception of dyspnea
5. Shared genetic factors
6. Shared life style factors
   - Diet
   - Decreased exercise
   - Sedentary lifestyle
7. Hormonal influences/puberty

Leptin, a product of the *ob* gene expressed predominantly in adipose tissue, is among the most studied proinflammatory adipokines. Serum levels of leptin are markedly increased in obesity. Leptin has effects on the innate and adaptive immune responses. Evidence suggests that high leptin levels are associated with higher asthma prevalence in prepubertal boys[39] and peri- and postpubertal girls.[40] High serum leptin concentrations are associated with increased severity of exercise-induced bronchoconstriction[41] and low peak expiratory flow rate[42] in children.

Adiponectin predominantly has antiinflammatory properties. It inhibits the production and effects of proinflammatory cytokines like tumor necrosis factor-α and IL-6. It induces the expression of antiinflammatory cytokines like IL-1 receptor antagonist and IL-10. However, it also exerts proinflammatory properties under certain conditions. Adiponectin levels are inversely related to BMI and obesity, and increase with weight loss.[38] Presence of adiponectin and receptors in lung suggest their possible role in the asthma–obesity link.

Animal studies have shown that adiponectin treatment markedly reduces allergen-induced airway inflammation and hyperresponsiveness.[43] Low serum adiponectin levels are associated with increased asthma prevalence and future risk of asthma in women.[44,45] High serum adiponectin levels have been associated with adverse clinical outcomes of asthma (more frequent active disease, frequent asthma medication use) in men but in not women.[46] A prospective study involving 368 urban adolescents with moderate to severe asthma showed that adiponectin levels were inversely related to severity of asthma status (asthma symptoms and exacerbations) and positively related to forced expiratory volume in 1 second (FEV_1)/forced vital capacity (FVC).[47] Serum adiponectin levels are also significantly negatively correlated with exercise-induced bronchoconstriction in children.[41]

Resistin is a proinflammatory adipokine, and derives its name from its ability to resist insulin ("resistance to insulin"). Few data are available on the role of resistin in asthma. One Korean study revealed that atopic childhood asthmatics had lower resistin levels compared with nonatopic asthmatics and control group.[48] It also demonstrated that resistin correlated positively with methacholine PC(20) and negatively with eosinophil count and total IgE. These findings suggest that resistin might have a protective role in asthma.

DOES CHILDHOOD OBESITY PROMOTE MIXED T HELPER CELL TYPE 1/2 INFLAMMATION?

Because adiposity is characterized by low-grade systemic inflammation, it is possible that adiposity influences allergic disorders through effects on the immune response. Individuals with allergic disorders usually have a T helper cell type 2 (Th2) polarization. A number of studies have tried to assess the Th polarization in obese subjects.

In a study involving obese asthmatic children, nonobese asthmatic children, obese nonasthmatic children, and nonobese nonasthmatic children, it was found that obese asthmatic children had significantly higher Th1 responses to a mitogen–phorbol 12-myristate 13-acetate and tetanus toxoid and lower Th2 responses to phorbol 12-myristate 13-acetate and *Dermatophagoides farinae* compared with nonobese asthmatic children.[49] Th cell patterns did not differ between obese asthmatic children and obese nonasthmatic children.[49] It is possible that adipokines skew the Th1/Th2 balance in favor of the Th1 response seen in asthma associated with obesity.[50,51] Further, this could also explain the reason for the poor association of obesity with other allergic disorders, which have a predominant Th2 response.

ARE OBESE CHILDREN AT HIGHER RISK OF HAVING AIRWAY HYPER-RESPONSIVENESS?

Airway hyperresponsiveness (AHR) is a characteristic feature of asthma. Many studies have been conducted in children and adults with conflicting evidence on the role of obesity in enhancing or modifying airway responsiveness. AHR has been assessed using methacholine, histamine, or exercise. Cross-sectional data analysis of the Childhood Asthma Management Program on 1039 US children aged 5 to 12 years suggested no effect of BMI on AHR after adjusting for baseline FEV_1.[32] A prospective birth cohort study from New Zealand on 1037 children followed for 26 years found no effect of BMI on AHR.[20] A Korean cross-sectional study found increased AHR in obese versus nonobese boys but not girls.[52] Likewise, a Taiwanese cross-sectional study on adolescents suggested that AHR increased with BMI, but only in girls.[21] All of these studies used methacholine as the bronchoconstricting agent. Even as AHR assessed using methacholine or histamine shows conflicting evidence, reports on exercise-induced bronchospasm are more consistent. These few small studies assessing exercise-induced bronchospasm have found greater severity of exercise-induced bronchospasm in obese versus nonobese children.[41,53]

LUNG FUNCTION IN OBESE ASTHMATICS

Increased body fat exerts direct mechanical effects on the respiratory system and reduces lung volumes. The most prominent and consistent effect of obesity is a reduction in expiratory reserve volume (ERV) and functional residual capacity (FRC). Evidence from a large adult study of 373 patients with normal FEV_1/FVC ratio, showed a consistent decline in all lung volumes (especially FRC and ERV) with an increase in BMI from 20 to 30 kg/m^2.[54]

Obese individuals breathe at low tidal volumes and high respiratory rate. Breathing at low FRC with low tidal volumes, decreases airway caliber, and thereby increases airway resistance. Lower FRC unloads the airway smooth muscle, which makes it liable to shorten more when stimulated by bronchoconstricting agents or parasympathetic tone.[43] It has also been observed that obese individuals breathe close to their closing volumes, making it prone to more frequent opening and closing, causing lung damage.

In contrast with the consistent observation for lung volumes in obese children, the effect of obesity on lung function is not consistent in studies. However, most studies show a decrease[32,47,55] or no change[26,56] in FEV_1/FVC ratio with increasing BMI. The conflicting studies in children could also be explained by the distribution of BMI among the participants. With a more normal distribution of BMI, lung function is likely to have a positive relationship with BMI. On the other hand, predominantly obese subjects with markedly high BMI are likely to have poorer lung function.

Spirometry parameters are affected by many factors, the most important of which are age, height, weight, gender, and race.[57] However, because it is lean muscle mass that is actually responsible for the increments in lung function rather than fat mass, BMI, which takes into account both lean and fat mass, may not be an appropriate surrogate of adiposity to assess a relationship between increasing fat mass and lung function. The effect of gender on the pattern of lung growth and fat deposition may be responsible for the differing patterns of lung function abnormalities seen in males and females.

OBESITY AND ASTHMA-RELATED OUTCOMES

Although many studies in adults have evaluated asthma-related outcomes (asthma control, severity, and exacerbations), pediatric data are limited. A large retrospective study of more than 32,000 US children and adolescents found increased usage of β-agonists and corticosteroids in obese/overweight asthmatics even after adjustment for confounders and comorbidities.[58] Similarly, data from the GALA II and SAGE II studies showed that poor asthma control was associated with increased BMI, but only in boys, who had a 33% greater chance of worse asthma control as compared with normal-weight boys.[59] Another prospective study of 368 adolescents with moderate-to-severe asthma demonstrated that high BMI was associated with poorer asthma control (increased symptom days and risk of exacerbation) in females only.[47] Obese asthmatics with acute, severe asthma admitted to pediatric intensive care units have been found to recover more slowly than the nonobese counterparts.[60]

On the other hand, a retrospective study found no difference in the usage of controller medications, steroid bursts, and FEV_1/FVC among different weight group asthmatic children (normal weight, overweight, and obese).[31] A prospective study evaluating 108 children and adolescents in a specialty asthma clinic found no association between obesity and asthma severity.[61]

To summarize, there is evidence to suggest that obese asthmatics have more symptoms, use quick relief medications more often, have poorly controlled asthma, and recover more slowly from acute exacerbations.

ROLE OF COMORBIDITIES

Obesity and asthma are both associated with certain comorbidities like SDB and GERD, which may be responsible, partly, for the said association between the two. There are few studies in children that have assessed the role and temporal relationship of these comorbidities in the obesity–asthma link.

A large, community-based study evaluated the relationship between obesity, SDB, and wheezing.[62] The authors demonstrated that both obesity and SDB were associated with wheeze/asthma. Another study demonstrated that SDB was associated with higher exhaled nitric oxide values in obese children compared with normal weight or overweight controls.[63]

GERD is associated with both asthma and obesity. Treatment of GERD is known to improve asthma control. Theoretically, GERD could partly explain the challenges of asthma control observed in obese individuals. A New Zealand birth cohort of 1037 individuals followed to 26 years of age found association of GERD with respiratory symptoms, independent of BMI.[20] Results from the European Community Respiratory Health Survey, which enrolled 2661 adults aged 20 to 48 years from 3 countries, found a strong association between nocturnal reflux symptoms and not only asthma and respiratory symptoms, but also obstructive sleep apnea[64]; the association was independent of BMI. A follow-up questionnaire survey of the European Community Respiratory Health Survey participants evaluated obesity, nocturnal reflux, and habitual snoring as risk factors for asthma onset.[65] The study demonstrated that onset of asthma, wheeze, and night-time symptoms were associated with obesity, nocturnal reflux, and habitual snoring.

To summarize, GERD and SDB are related to both obesity and asthma. However, the causality and temporal relationship of these comorbidities in the obesity–asthma link is not yet established.

WEIGHT LOSS AND ASTHMA CONTROL

The causal relation of obesity and incident asthma can be confirmed by the improvement in asthma outcomes with weight loss. A recent, small, prospective randomized controlled trial reported that weight reduction in obese individuals with severe uncontrolled asthma was associated with improved asthma control but no reduction in airway inflammation or bronchial hyperresponsiveness.[66] A study on weight loss using multidisciplinary intervention involving 76 obese adolescents (50 with and 26 without asthma) reported significant improvement in lung function.[67] The asthmatics demonstrated improvement in adiponectin levels, and reduction in C-reactive protein and leptin levels. Change in adiponectin emerged as an independent factor for improved lung function.

A systematic review evaluating weight loss and asthma demonstrated a consistent improvement in at least one asthma-related outcome in all 15 eligible studies.[68] Standard asthma management protocols now mention weight loss as a part of therapy in obese/overweight individuals.[69]

SUMMARY

Obesity affects different allergic diseases in different ways. The strongest association of obesity has been with nonallergic asthma compared with allergic asthma. Because eosinophilic inflammation has not been shown to increase in obese asthmatics, the mechanisms are likely to be other than augmentation of Th2 responses. The evidence of association with allergic diseases other than asthma is conflicting. The association is more consistent with eczema, but poor or inverse with allergic rhinitis/rhinoconjunctivitis, the conditions in which Th2 pathways play a major role. The association between asthma and obesity is also modified with comorbidities like SDB and GERD. The strength of association between asthma and obesity makes the need of weight loss as a part of standard asthma care and management.

REFERENCES

1. Akinbami LJ, Moorman JE, Garbe PL, et al. Status of childhood asthma in the United States: 1980-2007. Pediatrics 2009;123:S131–45.
2. Jackson KD, Howie LD, Akinbami LJ. Trends in allergic conditions among children: United States, 1997-2011. NCHS Data Brief 2013;(121):1–8.
3. Ogden CL, Carroll MD, Kit BK, et al. Prevalence of obesity and trends in body mass index among US children and adolescents, 1999-2010. JAMA 2012;307:483–90.
4. Castro-Rodríguez JA, Holberg CJ, Morgan WJ, et al. Increased incidence of asthmalike symptoms in girls who become overweight or obese during the school years. Am J Respir Crit Care Med 2001;163:1344–9.
5. Mannino DM, Mott J, Ferdinands JM, et al. Boys with high body masses have an increased risk of developing asthma: findings from the National Longitudinal Survey of Youth (NLSY). Int J Obes (Lond) 2006;30:6–13.
6. Gilliland FD, Berhane K, Islam T, et al. Obesity and the risk of newly diagnosed asthma in school-age children. Am J Epidemiol 2003;158:406–15.
7. Brumpton B, Langhammer A, Romundstad P, et al. General and abdominal obesity and incident asthma in adults: the HUNT study. Eur Respir J 2013;41:323–9.
8. Camargo CA Jr, Weiss ST, Zhang S, et al. Prospective study of body mass index, weight change, and risk of adult-onset asthma in women. Arch Intern Med 1999;159:2582–8.
9. Figueroa-Muñoz JI, Chinn S, Rona RJ. Association between obesity and asthma in 4-11 year old children in the UK. Thorax 2001;56:133–7.
10. von Kries R, Hermann M, Grunert VP, et al. Is obesity a risk factor for childhood asthma? Allergy 2001;56:318–22.

11. Kuschnir FC, da Cunha AL. Association of overweight with asthma prevalence in adolescents in Rio de Janeiro, Brazil. J Asthma 2009;46:928–32.
12. Mitchell EA, Beasley R, Björkstén B, et al, ISAAC Phase Three Study Group. The association between BMI, vigorous physical activity and television viewing and the risk of symptoms of asthma, rhinoconjunctivitis and eczema in children and adolescents: ISAAC Phase Three. Clin Exp Allergy 2013;43:73–84.
13. Black MH, Zhou H, Takayanagi M, et al. Increased asthma risk and asthma-related health care complications associated with childhood obesity. Am J Epidemiol 2013;178:1120–8.
14. von Mutius E, Schwartz J, Neas LM, et al. Relation of body mass index to asthma and atopy in children: the National Health and Nutrition Examination Study III. Thorax 2001;56:835–8.
15. Visness CM, London SJ, Daniels JL, et al. Association of childhood obesity with atopic and nonatopic asthma: results from the National Health and Nutrition Examination Survey 1999-2006. J Asthma 2010;47:822–9.
16. Jarvis D, Chinn S, Potts J, et al. European Community Respiratory Health Survey. Association of body mass index with respiratory symptoms and atopy: results from the European Community Respiratory Health Survey. Clin Exp Allergy 2002;32:831–7.
17. Garcia-Marcos L, Arnedo Pena A, Busquets-Monge R, et al. How the presence of rhinoconjunctivitis and the severity of asthma modify the relationship between obesity and asthma in children 6-7 years old. Clin Exp Allergy 2008;38:1174–8.
18. Silva MJ, Ribeiro MC, Carvalho F, et al. Atopic disease and body mass index. Allergol Immunopathol (Madr) 2007;35:130–5.
19. Schachter LM, Peat JK, Salome CM. Asthma and atopy in overweight children. Thorax 2003;58:1031–5.
20. Hancox RJ, Milne BJ, Poulton R, et al. Sex differences in the relation between body mass index and asthma and atopy in a birth cohort. Am J Respir Crit Care Med 2005;171:440–5.
21. Huang SL, Shiao G, Chou P. Association between body mass index and allergy in teenage girls in Taiwan. Clin Exp Allergy 1999;29:323–9.
22. Kusunoki T, Morimoto T, Nishikomori R, et al. Obesity and the prevalence of allergic diseases in schoolchildren. Pediatr Allergy Immunol 2008;19:527–34.
23. Silverberg JI, Kleiman E, Lev-Tov H, et al. Association between obesity and atopic dermatitis in childhood: a case-control study. J Allergy Clin Immunol 2011;127:1180–6.
24. Van Gysel D, Govaere E, Verhamme K, et al. Body mass index in Belgian schoolchildren and its relationship with sensitization and allergic symptoms. Pediatr Allergy Immunol 2009;20:246–53.
25. Fenger RV, Gonzalez-Quintela A, Vidal C, et al. Exploring the obesity-asthma link: do all types of adiposity increase the risk of asthma? Clin Exp Allergy 2012;42:1237–45.
26. Cibella F, Cuttitta G, La Grutta S, et al. A cross-sectional study assessing the relationship between BMI, asthma, atopy, and eNO among schoolchildren. Ann Allergy Asthma Immunol 2011;107:330–6.
27. Musaad SM, Patterson T, Ericksen M, et al. Comparison of anthropometric measures of obesity in childhood allergic asthma: central obesity is most relevant. J Allergy Clin Immunol 2009;123:1321–7.
28. Spathopoulos D, Paraskakis E, Trypsianis G, et al. The effect of obesity on pulmonary lung function of school aged children in Greece. Pediatr Pulmonol 2009; 44:273–80.

29. Chen Y, Rennie D, Cormier Y, et al. Atopy, obesity, and asthma in adults: the Humboldt study. J Agromedicine 2009;14:222–7.

30. Leung TF, Kong AP, Chan IH, et al. Association between obesity and atopy in Chinese schoolchildren. Int Arch Allergy Immunol 2009;149:133–40.

31. Ross KR, Storfer-Isser A, Hart MA, et al. Sleep-disordered breathing is associated with asthma severity in children. J Pediatr 2012;160:736–42.

32. Tantisira KG, Litonjua AA, Weiss ST, et al, Childhood Asthma Management Program Research Group. Association of body mass with pulmonary function in the Childhood Asthma Management Program (CAMP). Thorax 2003;58:1036–41.

33. Hasler G, Gergen PJ, Ajdacic V, et al. Asthma and body weight change: a 20-year prospective community study of young adults. Int J Obes (Lond) 2006;30:1111–8.

34. Green TL. Examining the temporal relationships between childhood obesity and asthma. Econ Hum Biol 2014;14:92–102.

35. Jensen ME, Wood LG, Gibson PG. Obesity and childhood asthma - mechanisms and manifestations. Curr Opin Allergy Clin Immunol 2012;12:186–92.

36. Boulet LP. Asthma and obesity. Clin Exp Allergy 2013;43:8–21.

37. Rasmussen F, Hancox RJ. Mechanisms of obesity in asthma. Curr Opin Allergy Clin Immunol 2014;14:35–43.

38. Sood A, Shore SA. Adiponectin, leptin, and resistin in asthma: basic mechanisms through Population Studies. J Allergy (Cairo) 2013;2013:785835.

39. Guler N, Kirerleri E, Ones U, et al. Leptin: does it have any role in childhood asthma? J Allergy Clin Immunol 2004;114:254–9.

40. Nagel G, Koenig W, Rapp K, et al. Associations of adipokines with asthma, rhinoconjunctivitis, and eczema in German schoolchildren. Pediatr Allergy Immunol 2009;20:81–8.

41. Baek HS, Kim YD, Shin JH, et al. Serum leptin and adiponectin levels correlate with exercise-induced bronchoconstriction in children with asthma. Ann Allergy Asthma Immunol 2011;107:14–21.

42. Gurkan F, Atamer Y, Ece A, et al. Serum leptin levels in asthmatic children treated with an inhaled corticosteroid. Ann Allergy Asthma Immunol 2004;93:277–80.

43. Shore SA, Johnston RA. Obesity and asthma. Pharmacol Ther 2006;110:83–102.

44. Sood A, Cui X, Qualls C, et al. Association between asthma and serum adiponectin concentration in women. Thorax 2008;63:877–82.

45. Sood A, Qualls C, Schuyler M, et al. Low serum adiponectin predicts future risk for asthma in women. Am J Respir Crit Care Med 2012;186:41–7.

46. Sood A, Dominic E, Qualls C, et al. Serum adiponectin is associated with adverse outcomes of asthma in men but not in women. Front Pharmacol 2011;2:55.

47. Kattan M, Kumar R, Bloomberg GR, et al. Asthma control, adiposity, and adipokines among inner-city adolescents. J Allergy Clin Immunol 2010;125:584–92.

48. Kim KW, Shin YH, Lee KE, et al. Relationship between adipokines and manifestations of childhood asthma. Pediatr Allergy Immunol 2008;19:535–40.

49. Rastogi D, Canfield SM, Andrade A, et al. Obesity-associated asthma in children: a distinct entity. Chest 2012;141:895–905.

50. Tilg H, Moschen AR. Adipocytokines: mediators linking adipose tissue, inflammation and immunity. Nat Rev Immunol 2006;6:772–83.

51. Baumann S, Lorentz A. Obesity - a promoter of allergy? Int Arch Allergy Immunol 2013;162:205–13.

52. Jang AS, Lee JH, Park SW, et al. Severe airway hyperresponsiveness in school-aged boys with a high body mass index. Korean J Intern Med 2006;21:10–4.
53. Lopes WA, Radominski RB, Rosário Filho NA, et al. Exercise-induced broncho-spasm in obese adolescents. Allergol Immunopathol (Madr) 2009;37:175–9.
54. Jones RL, Nzekwu MM. The effects of body mass index on lung volumes. Chest 2006;130:827–33.
55. Lang JE, Hossain J, Smith K, et al. Asthma severity, exacerbation risk, and controller treatment burden in underweight and obese children. J Asthma 2012;49:456–63.
56. Peters JI, McKinney JM, Smith B, et al. Impact of obesity in asthma: evidence from a large prospective disease management study. Ann Allergy Asthma Immunol 2011;106:30–5.
57. Quanjer PH, Stanojevic S, Cole TJ, et al. ERS global lung function initiative. Multi-ethnic reference values for spirometry for the 3-95-yr age range: the global lung function 2012 equations. Eur Respir J 2012;40:1324–43.
58. Quinto KB, Zuraw BL, Poon KY, et al. The association of obesity and asthma severity and control in children. J Allergy Clin Immunol 2011;128:964–9.
59. Borrell LN, Nguyen EA, Roth LA, et al. Childhood obesity and asthma control in the GALA II and SAGE II studies. Am J Respir Crit Care Med 2013;187:697–702.
60. Giese JK. Pediatric obesity and its effects on asthma control. J Am Assoc Nurse Pract 2014;26:102–9.
61. Carroll CL, Bhandari A, Zucker AR, et al. Childhood obesity increases duration of therapy during severe asthma exacerbations. Pediatr Crit Care Med 2006;7:527–31.
62. Sulit LG, Storfer-Isser A, Rosen CL, et al. Associations of obesity, sleep-disordered breathing, and wheezing in children. Am J Respir Crit Care Med 2005;171:659–64.
63. Verhulst SL, Aerts L, Jacobs S, et al. Sleep-disordered breathing, obesity, and airway inflammation in children and adolescents. Chest 2008;134:1169–75.
64. Gislason T, Janson C, Vermeire P, et al. Respiratory symptoms and nocturnal gastroesophageal reflux: a population-based study of young adults in three European countries. Chest 2002;121:158–63.
65. Gunnbjörnsdóttir MI, Omenaas E, Gíslason T, et al, RHINE Study Group. Obesity and nocturnal gastro-oesophageal reflux are related to onset of asthma and respiratory symptoms. Eur Respir J 2004;24:116–21.
66. Dias-Júnior SA, Reis M, de Carvalho-Pinto RM, et al. Effects of weight loss on asthma control in obese patients with severe asthma. Eur Respir J 2014;43(5):1368–77.
67. da Silva PL, de Mello MT, Cheik NC, et al. Interdisciplinary therapy improves biomarkers profile and lung function in asthmatic obese adolescents. Pediatr Pulmonol 2012;47:8–17.
68. Eneli IU, Skybo T, Camargo CA Jr. Weight loss and asthma: a systematic review. Thorax 2008;63:671–6.
69. Global Initiative for Asthma. Global Strategy for Asthma Management and Prevention: 2012 update. Available at: http://www.ginasthma.org/local/uploads/files/GINA_Report_March13.pdf. Accessed January 20, 2014.

Arginine Metabolism in Asthma

Jeremy A. Scott, PhD[a], Hartmut Grasemann, MD, PhD[b],*

KEYWORDS

- Arginine metabolism • Nitric oxide synthase • Arginase • Agmatine • Citrulline
- Ornithine • Polyamine • ADMA

KEY POINTS

- L-Arginine metabolism via the arginase and nitric oxide synthase pathways is important in maintenance of airways muscular tone.
- Imbalance in the L-arginine metabolism leading to nitric oxide deficiency and airway constriction can occur through increased arginase activity or by accumulation of endogenous nitric oxide synthase inhibitors such as asymmetric dimethylarginine (ADMA).
- ADMA may represent a novel therapeutic target in correcting the enhanced airways responsiveness in asthma.

INTRODUCTION

The semiessential amino acid, L-arginine, serves many functions in cellular and organ homeostasis. Of particular relevance to physiologic function is the production of nitric oxide (NO) from L-arginine by the nitric oxide synthase (NOS) family of isozymes, which serves to relax airway smooth muscle cells through direct interaction with the heme core of soluble guanylate cyclase. The production of NO can be modified in disease by increased competition between NOS and the arginase pathway, which produces urea and ornithine. The authors, and other investigators, have previously reported that the airways hypercontractility in animal models of asthma is at least in part related to imbalances in the production of NO by the neuronal NOS,[1] as well as increased competition for substrate L-arginine with the arginases.[2–4] It has more recently become appreciated that the production of the endogenous NOS inhibitor, asymmetric dimethylarginine (ADMA), as well as accumulation of the L-ornithine–derived

[a] Division of Biomedical Sciences, Department of Health Sciences, Faculty of Health and Behavioural Sciences, Northern Ontario School of Medicine, Lakehead University, 955 Oliver Road Thunder Bay, Ontario P7B 5E1, Canada; [b] Program in Physiology and Experimental Medicine, Research Institute, and Division of Respiratory Medicine, Department of Pediatrics, The Hospital for Sick Children, University of Toronto, 555 University Avenue, Toronto, Ontario M5G 1X8, Canada
* Corresponding author.
E-mail address: hartmut.grasemann@sickkids.ca

Immunol Allergy Clin N Am 34 (2014) 767–775
http://dx.doi.org/10.1016/j.iac.2014.07.007
0889-8561/14/$ – see front matter © 2014 Elsevier Inc. All rights reserved.

polyamines, downstream of the arginase pathway, may also modify NO production and airway tone in asthma.[5,6]

ADMA in the Lung

Synthesis of ADMA (protein arginine methyltransferases)

The first step of arginine incorporation into proteins is through the attachment of arginine to the corresponding transfer RNA (tRNA) anticodon via aminoacyl tRNA synthetase. The arginine residue is inserted into the forming protein by the ribosomal complex and the formation of a peptide bond. Methyl groups are then added to the arginine residues in proteins by a family of protein arginine methyltransferases (PRMTs).[7] The 2 classes of PRMTs, type I and II, exhibit differential kinetics for the formation of asymmetric (ADMA) versus symmetric dimethylarginine (SDMA), respectively, in addition to synthesis of monomethyl arginine (MMA).[7] Yildirim and colleagues[8] (2006) reported that PRMTs are expressed in the mouse lung within the bronchiolar and alveolar epithelium and that PRMT2 can be induced by chronic hypoxia. Bulau and colleagues[9] subsequently reported a comprehensive expression profile of the PRMTs in mouse lung and demonstrated expression of both type I (PRMT1, PRMT3, PRMT4, PRMT6) and type II PRMTs (PRMT5, PRMT7). Although alterations in PRMT expression have not yet been demonstrated in human asthma, Ahmad and colleagues[10,11] reported increased expression of PRMT2 protein levels in bronchial epithelium from their mouse model of ovalbumin (OVA)-induced allergic airways inflammation. Sun and colleagues[12,13] also comprehensively examined PRMT expression in their rat OVA model of allergic airways inflammation and demonstrated significant upregulation of PRMT1, PRMT2, and PRMT3 and downregulation of PRMT4 in the lungs. PRMT1 expression was quantified in immunostained sections and shown to be upregulated in the bronchi and alveolar epithelial cells. They further demonstrated that administration of an arginine methyltransferase inhibitor (AM-1) before the OVA exposure led to a reduction in inflammation, as assessed by eosinophil cell counts from bronchoalveolar lavage (BAL) fluid, semiquantitative scoring of histologic sections of the lungs, interleukin 4 (IL-4) messenger RNA expression, and quantification of immunoglobulin (Ig) E and OVA-specific IgG1 in serum.[13] Given the timing of the AM-1 inhibitor administration, the investigators posited that IL-4 induced PRMT1 expression, which led to the expression of eotaxin in the inflamed airways. Given the complex interaction of PRMTs with arginine metabolism, it would be very interesting to examine the changes in ADMA and the pathophysiologic/functional impact of administration of AM-1 in established disease (ie, is PRMT a good candidate for therapeutic intervention in asthma?). The role of altered expression of PRMTs and the impact on protein and physiologic functions in asthma is clearly an area that requires further investigation.

ADMA, SDMA, and MMA are liberated on proteolytic cleavage of proteins, allowing access of these derivates to the intracellular milieu. SDMA has been reported to inhibit the cationic amino acid transporters (CAT1, *SLC7A1*; CAT2, *SLC7A2*), which are the primary means of cellular uptake of L-arginine.[14,15] In addition to competition at the cationic amino acid transporters, MMA and ADMA also act directly as competitive inhibitors of NOS.[16] The accumulation of these endogenous NOS inhibitors likely leads to impaired NOS function, despite the presence of "normal" levels of L-arginine; this has been described as the "arginine paradox".[16]

Degradation of ADMA

ADMA is metabolically degraded to L-citrulline and dimethylamine by dimethylarginine dimethylaminohydrolases (DDAH).[17,18] The 2 members of this family of enzymes, DDAH1 and DDAH2, are differentially expressed in tissues, including the kidney, liver, lung, and heart. Bulau and colleagues[9] reported that DDAH1 was expressed at low levels, and DDAH2 was expressed at high levels in lungs from normal mice; however, DDAH enzymatic conversion of ADMA to L-citrulline was the highest in liver and kidney, suggesting a significant potential for circulating ADMA derived from the lung to manifest systemic effects. By contrast, SDMA is not metabolized appreciably in vivo, with heart, lung, kidneys, and liver being tested by Bulau and colleagues,[9] supporting its predominant renal excretion on liberation.

Klein and colleagues[19] (2010) reported that DDAH1-overexpressing transgenic mice exhibit an attenuated OVA-induced increase in pulmonary inflammation compared with wild-type controls. This effect on allergic airways inflammation was recently corroborated by Kinker and colleagues[20] (2014) using a house dust mite model in DDAH1-overexpressing mice, in which the attenuation of BAL inflammatory cells was completely attributable to a reduction in eosinophils, but not neutrophils. However, although Kinker and colleagues[20] reported decreased expression of both DDAH1 and DDAH2, the authors demonstrated that DDAH enzyme activity was altered neither in the acute OVA-induced allergic airways inflammation model in mice nor in lung tissue from human asthma.[5] Thus, the rate-limiting factor of ADMA metabolism in asthma would appear to be the presence of functional DDAH.

Additional evidence supporting an important role of DDAH in lung disease has also been shown in a mouse model of acute lung injury. Aggarwal and colleagues[21] recently reported that overexpression of DDAH2 in a mouse model of acute lung injury led to a reduction in ADMA levels as well as indices of oxidative/nitrosative stress in lungs and ameliorated the lung leak, injury, and functional changes following treatment with E. coli lipopolysaccharide (LPS). Thus, modification of ADMA metabolism by DDAH represents a potential therapeutic target in both bacteria- and allergy-induced pulmonary inflammation.

Functional Consequences of ADMA Liberation in the Lung

ADMA in vitro

Wells and Holian[22] (2007) reported that ADMA treatment of LA-4 lung epithelial (adenoma) cells, which had been primed with an LPS exposure, led to the production of reactive nitrogen and oxygen species, thus contributing to overall oxidative stress in these cells. These data suggested that ADMA may play an important role in airway inflammation and led to in vivo studies of allergic airways inflammation.

Animal studies

Wells and colleagues[23] (2009) furthermore treated normal BALB/c mice with ADMA via osmotic pump to achieve a chronic (2-week) systemic exposure and demonstrated increased total respiratory resistance and reduced dynamic compliance, thus evidencing altered lung function in response to ADMA. These changes were attributed to increased collagen production via the arginase pathway, leading to increased levels of hydroxyproline, a precursor for collagen biosynthesis. Interestingly, these changes in respiratory function were reversed after withdrawal of ADMA for 4 weeks, supporting the potential therapeutic benefit of targeting this pathway. They further demonstrated increased arginase enzyme activity with ADMA, both in vitro and in vivo, in the absence of increased expression of arginase. They posited that this increase was due to disinhibition of arginase by the lack of production of the intermediate of the NOS biosynthetic pathway NO-hydroxy-arginine, which inhibits arginase. Klein and colleagues[19] (2010) went on to demonstrate that exogenous systemic ADMA (also delivered by osmotic pump) further augmented pulmonary eosinophilic and neutrophilic inflammation in the OVA model of allergic airways inflammation.

Consistent with the findings of Wells and colleagues[23] and Ahmad and colleagues,[10] the authors reported elevated levels of both ADMA and SDMA in an acute model of OVA-induced allergic airways inflammation.[5] These observations were extended to demonstrate increased airways contractility to methacholine in response to the acute administration of levels of ADMA similar to those observed in the model mice, thus demonstrating that ADMA at levels observed in the OVA model could achieve the degree of airway hyperresponsiveness observed in disease.[5]

Recently the ratio of L-arginine:ADMA has been postulated in the cardiovascular literature to explain what is called the "arginine paradox", the apparent dysfunction of NOS activity even in the presence of "normal" levels of L-arginine.[16] As such, the normal L-arginine:ADMA ratio would be in the 100 to 200 range, with attenuation indicated in the presence of cardiovascular disease.[16] Bulau and colleagues[9] (2007) reported similar L-arginine:ADMA ratios in BAL and serum from control mice and human subjects (range: 108 ± 20 and 163 ± 26 for BAL from mice and humans, respectively; and 124 ± 14 and 166 ± 29 for serum from mice and humans, respectively), thus supporting that peripheral indices of L-arginine:ADMA changes reflect alterations within the lungs in both species. Interestingly, the authors demonstrated similar ratios in normal mice and human tissues, which were attenuated in their mice with allergic airways inflammation and in human asthma.[5]

Ahmad and colleagues[10] (2010) reported increased ADMA levels in their OVA model of allergic airways inflammation, with concomitant elevation of peroxynitrite and nitrotyrosine levels in mitochondria and lung cytosol, respectively. Ahmad and colleagues[10] further demonstrated increased bronchial epithelial cell expression of PRMT2 and decreased expression of DDAH2 by Western blotting and immunohistochemical staining. Ahmad and colleagues[11] (2011) subsequently reported that simvastatin administration during the allergen challenge phase of the acute OVA model led to induction of endothelial NOS expression and attenuation of inducible NOS expression, apoptosis, inflammation, and Th2 cytokines (IL-4, IL-5, IL-13) and more importantly that the augmented methacholine responsiveness in these mice was attenuated compared with the vehicle-treated OVA-inflamed mice.

Increased arginase activity results in increased production of proline, a precursor of collagen, and formation of the L-ornithine–derived polyamines putrescine, spermidine and spermine. Inhibition of NOS and increased L-arginine:ADMA ratio may result in increased consumption of L-arginine by arginase and increased formation of polyamines. The authors have observed increased polyamines in mouse lungs from the acute OVA-induced allergic airways inflammation model.[24] The importance of this observation lies in the role of spermine as an inhibitor of NOS, because nebulization of spermine into mouse airways resulted in a decrease in NO formation and increase in airway hyperresponsiveness to methacholine.[24]

Clinical studies

The authors reported that ADMA levels were elevated 2.4-fold in sputum from pediatric patients with asthma compared with control subjects. Sputum ADMA levels and L-arginine:ADMA ratios correlated significantly with fractional exhaled NO (FeNO) in the patients with asthma, suggesting physiologic relevance of ADMA as NOS inhibitor in human asthma airways. Similarly, the L-arginine:ADMA ratios were also significantly reduced in asthma lung tissues compared with control lung tissues, matching the observation in mouse lung tissue.[5]

Increased levels of ADMA were also found in exhaled breath condensate (EBC) from children with asthma. There was no significant difference in EBC ADMA between children treated or not treated with inhaled corticosteroids. In this study, there were no significant correlations between EBC ADMA with serum ADMA levels, FeNO, or lung function parameters.[5,25]

Further evidence of a potential role of ADMA in airway responsiveness comes from a study of adult patients with mild, eosinophilic asthma where ADMA was measured in induced sputum before and after a controlled inhaled allergen challenge. Sputum ADMA was increased significantly in these patients 7 and 24 hours after the challenge, along with increases in sputum eosinophils and changes in pulmonary function testing consistent with airflow limitation and airway hyperresponsiveness.[26]

Seemingly conflicting data exist in regards to systemic levels of ADMA in asthma. In a case-control study of 50 pediatric patients with mild allergic asthma, FeNO was found to be increased, as expected, whereas mean plasma ADMA and L-arginine concentrations were significantly lower than in healthy controls.[27] Although the reduced systemic L-arginine concentrations confirmed results of an earlier study by Morris and colleagues in a mixed population of pediatric and adult patients with asthma, and may be explained by increased concentrations of free arginase in blood, low circulating levels of ADMA and L-arginine were not confirmed in a cohort of 8-year-old children with asthma. However, the patients in this particular study had very mild asthma, were no different in post-bronchodilator spirometry (forced expiratory volume in the first second of expiration [FEV_1], forced vital capacity [FVC], or FEV_1/FVC) from their age-matched nonasthmatic controls, and did not have increased mean FeNO.[28]

There is growing evidence that obesity is associated with the development of asthma.[29,30] Obesity is an important factor among female patients whose asthma occurs after childhood and who have less atopy, using cluster analyses,[31,32] and this cluster was also associated with lower airway eosinophils and FeNO.[32,33] The inverse association between body mass index (BMI) and FeNO[34] may be explained by an imbalance between L-arginine and ADMA, because ADMA concentration and the L-arginine:ADMA ratio in plasma were reported to have similar associations with FeNO as for sputum among late onset asthma.[6,35,36] Specifically, subjects with late-onset asthma had higher ADMA and lower L-arginine plasma levels compared with early onset, respectively. The log plasma L-arginine:ADMA ratio was inversely correlated with BMI in late-onset but not the early-onset asthma. Although FeNO was inversely associated with BMI in the late-onset phenotype, the relationship was lost after adjusting for L-arginine:ADMA ratio. Also in this phenotype, a reduced L-arginine:ADMA ratio was associated with less serum IgE, increased respiratory symptoms, lower lung volumes, and worse asthma quality of life.[6]

These studies not only provided evidence that ADMA may be a link between obesity and asthma, but also demonstrated that clinical-biological phenotyping in asthma may help unravel pathways beyond inflammation that lead to asthma and potentially to new asthma treatments.[37]

TREATMENT OPTIONS

As both animal and human studies suggested that the L-arginine:ADMA ratio is important in the development of NO-mediated airway hyperresponsiveness and asthma, therapies that would result in increased availability of L-arginine for NOS could potentially be beneficial in asthma.

Mabalirajan and colleagues[38] examined the effect of a high dose of L-arginine (250 mg/kg, twice daily) on airway hyperresponsiveness in the mouse OVA-model of allergic airways inflammation and demonstrated a reduction of the methacholine-induced airways resistance changes in treated mice compared with untreated

OVA-stimulated animals. Interestingly, the high-dose L-arginine treatment also led to a reduction of pulmonary arginase activity, which might be attributable to increased production of the arginase inhibitor N^{ω}-hydroxy-L-arginine as an intermediate metabolite of the NOS pathway. Administration of high-dose L-arginine also further augmented expired NO from the allergically inflamed mice, which reinforces the role of the different compartments within the lungs, airways, and infiltrating inflammatory cells in the disease pathogenesis.

Supplementation with L-arginine should theoretically improve the L-arginine:ADMA ratio but the effectiveness of this approach may be limited by the high first-pass mechanism of L-arginine in the gut and liver. In addition, recent clinical trials have suggested that long-term supplementation with this amino acid may also result in an increase in ADMA formation.[39,40] Delivery of L-citrulline, which serves a substrate for *de novo* synthesis of L-arginine, may help circumvent some of these problems as L-citrulline supplementation has been shown to lead to increased L-arginine levels and beneficial effects in heart failure and sepsis.[41,42]

However, as arginase is upregulated in asthma,[2,4,43] strategies that increase L-arginine concentrations may ultimately result in increased arginase activity and the formation of polyamines and proline. The polyamine spermine was recently shown to contribute to airway hyperresponsiveness in asthma by inhibiting NOS,[24] and proline may contribute to airway remodeling, because it is a precursor of collagen formation.[24,44,45] Therefore, arginase inhibition may be a more elegant approach than L-arginine or L-citrulline supplementation, because it would result not only in an increase in

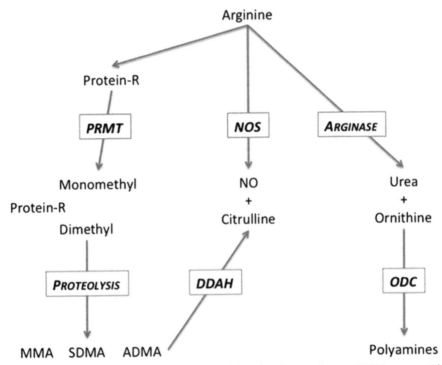

Fig. 1. Metabolism of L-arginine via the PRMT, NOS, and arginase pathways. ADMA, asymmetric dimethylarginine; DDAH, dimethylarginine dimethylaminohydrolases; MMA, monomethylarginine; NO, nitric oxide; NOS, nitric oxide synthase; ODC, ornithine decarboxylase; PRMT, protein arginine methyltransferases; SDMA, symmetric dimethylarginine.

L-arginine availability for NOS but also a decrease in the production of factors that contribute to airway remodeling.[2,46,47]

Future strategies may include a reduction of ADMA synthesis by inhibiting PRMTs or enhancing metabolic breakdown by increasing the enzymatic activity of DDAH.

FUTURE CONSIDERATIONS/SUMMARY

Current evidence suggests that L-arginine metabolism is altered in asthma. Changes in the balance of the L-arginine metabolism result in reduced L-arginine availability for NOS and impairment of the enzyme, which has significant functional consequences. Further studies will have to elucidate the role of other L-arginine metabolizing enzymes, including the arginine decarboxylase-agmatine-agmatinase pathway. A better characterization of the L-arginine metabolome in well-phenotyped patient populations may lead to a better understanding of the pathways involved and may offer new targets for therapeutic interventions (**Fig. 1**).

REFERENCES

1. De Sanctis GT, MacLean JA, Hamada K, et al. Contribution of nitric oxide synthases 1, 2, and 3 to airway hyperresponsiveness and inflammation in a murine model of asthma. J Exp Med 1999;189:1621–30.
2. North ML, Khanna N, Marsden PA, et al. Functionally important role for arginase 1 in the airway hyperresponsiveness of asthma. Am J Physiol Lung Cell Mol Physiol 2009;296:L911–20.
3. Meurs H, McKay S, Maarsingh H, et al. Increased arginase activity underlies allergen-induced deficiency of cnos-derived nitric oxide and airway hyperresponsiveness. Br J Pharmacol 2002;136:391–8.
4. Zimmermann N, King NE, Laporte J, et al. Dissection of experimental asthma with DNA microarray analysis identifies arginase in asthma pathogenesis. J Clin Invest 2003;111:1863–74.
5. Scott JA, North ML, Rafii M, et al. Asymmetric dimethylarginine is increased in asthma. Am J Respir Crit Care Med 2011;184:779–85.
6. Holguin F, Comhair SA, Hazen SL, et al. An association between l-arginine/asymmetric dimethyl arginine balance, obesity, and the age of asthma onset phenotype. Am J Respir Crit Care Med 2013;187:153–9.
7. Zakrzewicz D, Eickelberg O. From arginine methylation to adma: a novel mechanism with therapeutic potential in chronic lung diseases. BMC Pulm Med 2009;9:5.
8. Yildirim AO, Bulau P, Zakrzewicz D, et al. Increased protein arginine methylation in chronic hypoxia: role of protein arginine methyltransferases. Am J Respir Cell Mol Biol 2006;35:436–43.
9. Bulau P, Zakrzewicz D, Kitowska K, et al. Analysis of methylarginine metabolism in the cardiovascular system identifies the lung as a major source of adma. Am J Physiol Lung Cell Mol Physiol 2007;292:L18–24.
10. Ahmad T, Mabalirajan U, Ghosh B, et al. Altered asymmetric dimethyl arginine metabolism in allergically inflamed mouse lungs. Am J Respir Cell Mol Biol 2010;42:3–8.
11. Ahmad T, Mabalirajan U, Sharma A, et al. Simvastatin improves epithelial dysfunction and airway hyperresponsiveness: from asymmetric dimethyl-arginine to asthma. Am J Respir Cell Mol Biol 2011;44:531–9.
12. Sun QZ, Jiao FF, Yang XD, et al. Expression of protein arginine n-methyltransferases in e3 rat models of acute asthma. Nan Fang Yi Ke Da Xue Xue Bao 2010;30:716–9 [in Chinese].

13. Sun Q, Yang X, Zhong B, et al. Upregulated protein arginine methyltransferase 1 by il-4 increases eotaxin-1 expression in airway epithelial cells and participates in antigen-induced pulmonary inflammation in rats. J Immunol 2012;188:3506–12.

14. Closs EI, Basha FZ, Habermeier A, et al. Interference of l-arginine analogues with l-arginine transport mediated by the y+ carrier hcat-2B. Nitric Oxide 1997;1: 65–73.

15. Strobel J, Mieth M, Endress B, et al. Interaction of the cardiovascular risk marker asymmetric dimethylarginine (ADMA) with the human cationic amino acid transporter 1 (cat1). J Mol Cell Cardiol 2012;53:392–400.

16. Bode-Boger SM, Scalera F, Ignarro LJ. The L-arginine paradox: importance of the l-arginine/asymmetrical dimethylarginine ratio. Pharmacol Ther 2007;114: 295–306.

17. Pope AJ, Karrupiah K, Kearns PN, et al. Role of dimethylarginine dimethylamino-hydrolases in the regulation of endothelial nitric oxide production. J Biol Chem 2009;284:35338–47.

18. Pope AJ, Karuppiah K, Cardounel AJ. Role of the prmt-ddah-adma axis in the regulation of endothelial nitric oxide production. Pharmacol Res 2009;60: 461–5.

19. Klein E, Weigel J, Buford MC, et al. Asymmetric dimethylarginine potentiates lung inflammation in a mouse model of allergic asthma. Am J Physiol Lung Cell Mol Physiol 2010;299:L816–25.

20. Kinker KG, Gibson AM, Bass SA, et al. Overexpression of dimethylarginine dimethylaminohydrolase 1 attenuates airway inflammation in a mouse model of asthma. PLoS One 2014;9:e85148.

21. Aggarwal S, Gross CM, Kumar S, et al. Dimethylarginine dimethylaminohydrolase ii overexpression attenuates LPS-mediated lung leak in acute lung injury. Am J Respir Cell Mol Biol 2014;50:614–25.

22. Wells SM, Holian A. Asymmetric dimethylarginine induces oxidative and nitrosative stress in murine lung epithelial cells. Am J Respir Cell Mol Biol 2007;36: 520–8.

23. Wells SM, Buford MC, Migliaccio CT, et al. Elevated asymmetric dimethylarginine alters lung function and induces collagen deposition in mice. Am J Respir Cell Mol Biol 2009;40:179–88.

24. North ML, Grasemann H, Khanna N, et al. Increased ornithine-derived polyamines cause airway hyperresponsiveness in a mouse model of asthma. Am J Respir Cell Mol Biol 2013;48:694–702.

25. Carraro S, Giordano G, Piacentini G, et al. Asymmetric dimethylarginine in exhaled breath condensate and serum of children with asthma. Chest 2013; 144:405–10.

26. Scott JA, Gauvreau GM, Grasemann H. Asymmetric dimethylarginine and asthma. Eur Respir J 2014;43:647–8.

27. Riccioni G, Bucciarelli V, Verini M, et al. Adma, sdma, l-arginine and nitric oxide in allergic pediatric bronchial asthma. J Biol Regul Homeost Agents 2012;26:561–6.

28. Lau EM, Morgan PE, Belousova EG, et al. Asymmetric dimethylarginine and asthma: results from the childhood asthma prevention study. Eur Respir J 2013;41:1234–7.

29. Gonzalez JR, Caceres A, Esko T, et al. A common 16p11.2 inversion underlies the joint susceptibility to asthma and obesity. Am J Hum Genet 2014;94:361–72.

30. Kim HY, Lee HJ, Chang YJ, et al. Interleukin-17-producing innate lymphoid cells and the nlrp3 inflammasome facilitate obesity-associated airway hyperreactivity. Nat Med 2014;20:54–61.

31. Moore WC, Meyers DA, Wenzel SE, et al, National Heart Lung, Blood Institute's Severe Asthma Research Program. Identification of asthma phenotypes using cluster analysis in the severe asthma research program. Am J Respir Crit Care Med 2010;181:315–23.
32. Haldar P, Pavord ID, Shaw DE, et al. Cluster analysis and clinical asthma phenotypes. Am J Respir Crit Care Med 2008;178:218–24.
33. Sutherland ER, Goleva E, King TS, et al, Asthma Clinical Research Network. Cluster analysis of obesity and asthma phenotypes. PLoS One 2012;7:e36631.
34. Komakula S, Khatri S, Mermis J, et al. Body mass index is associated with reduced exhaled nitric oxide and higher exhaled 8-isoprostanes in asthmatics. Respir Res 2007;8:32.
35. Holguin F, Bleecker ER, Busse WW, et al. Obesity and asthma: an association modified by age of asthma onset. J Allergy Clin Immunol 2011;127:1486–93.e2.
36. Holguin F. Arginine and nitric oxide pathways in obesity-associated asthma. J Allergy (Cairo) 2013;2013:714595.
37. Sterk PJ, Ricciardolo FL. Clinical-biological phenotyping beyond inflammation in asthma delivers. Am J Respir Crit Care Med 2013;187:117–8.
38. Mabalirajan U, Ahmad T, Leishangthem GD, et al. Beneficial effects of high dose of l-arginine on airway hyperresponsiveness and airway inflammation in a murine model of asthma. J Allergy Clin Immunol 2010;125:626–35.
39. Grasemann H, Tullis E, Ratjen F. A randomized controlled trial of inhaled l-arginine in patients with cystic fibrosis. J Cyst Fibros 2013;12:468–74.
40. Kenyon NJ, Last M, Bratt JM, et al. L-arginine supplementation and metabolism in asthma. Pharmaceuticals 2011;4:187–201.
41. Balderas-Munoz K, Castillo-Martinez L, Orea-Tejeda A, et al. Improvement of ventricular function in systolic heart failure patients with oral l-citrulline supplementation. Cardiol J 2012;19:612–7.
42. Wijnands KA, Vink H, Briede JJ, et al. Citrulline a more suitable substrate than arginine to restore no production and the microcirculation during endotoxemia. PLoS One 2012;7:e37439.
43. Morris CR, Poljakovic M, Lavrisha L, et al. Decreased arginine bioavailability and increased serum arginase activity in asthma. Am J Respir Crit Care Med 2004; 170:148–53.
44. Sousse LE, Yamamoto Y, Enkhbaatar P, et al. Acute lung injury-induced collagen deposition is associated with elevated asymmetric dimethylarginine and arginase activity. Shock 2011;35:282–8.
45. Tanaka H, Masuda T, Tokuoka S, et al. The effect of allergen-induced airway inflammation on airway remodeling in a murine model of allergic asthma. Inflamm Res 2001;50:616–24.
46. Prado CM, Martins MA, Tiberio IF. Nitric oxide in asthma physiopathology. ISRN Allergy 2011;2011:832560.
47. Zeki AA, Bratt JM, Rabowsky M, et al. Simvastatin inhibits goblet cell hyperplasia and lung arginase in a mouse model of allergic asthma: a novel treatment for airway remodeling? Transl Res 2010;156:335–49.

Metabolic Asthma
Is There a Link Between Obesity, Diabetes, and Asthma?

Miriam K. Perez, MD, Giovanni Piedimonte, MD*

KEYWORDS

- Body mass index • Fetal programming • Lung development • Metabolic syndrome

KEY POINTS

- Regardless of body mass index percentile, children diagnosed with asthma are more likely to have higher triglyceride and insulin blood levels than children without asthma.
- Dyslipidemia and hyperinsulinemia, known silent precursors to cardiovascular disease, are also associated with the development of asthma, and confound its epidemiologic link to obesity.
- Diet and physical exercise may influence the development and persistence of innate and adaptive immune mechanisms involved in the pathogenesis of asthma in children.
- Prenatal events, such as intrauterine exposure to imbalanced maternal nutrition, may cause a shift in the trajectory of structural and functional airway development toward a hyperreactive phenotype.
- Monitoring and dietary/pharmacologic control of triglyceride and glucose metabolism during pregnancy and in the first years of life may become an important component of the prevention and management of asthma.

Childhood obesity has reached epidemic proportions worldwide, prompting First Lady Michelle Obama to launch the "Let's Move!" campaign against childhood obesity in February 2010.[1] Overweight is currently defined as a body mass index (BMI; calculated as the weight in kilograms divided by the height meters squared) from the 85th up to the 95th percentile for age, whereas obesity is defined as a BMI at or greater than the 95th percentile (**Fig. 1**).[2] Data from the Centers for Disease Control and Prevention (CDC) indicate that nearly 1 in 3 children in America are overweight or obese and that the rate of obesity already exceeds 30% in the United States.[3]

What is especially concerning is the rate at which this problem is growing. During the past 3 decades, childhood obesity rates in America have tripled.[4] Furthermore,

The authors have nothing to disclose.
Pediatric Institute and Children's Hospital, Cleveland Clinic, Cleveland, OH 44195, USA
* Corresponding author. Pediatric Institute and Children's Hospital, Cleveland Clinic, 9500 Euclid Avenue, A-111, Cleveland, OH 44195.
E-mail address: PIEDIMG@ccf.org

BMI= Weight/Height²
- Reliable indicator of overweight and obesity
- Easily obtained
- Strongly correlated with body fat percentage

- **Underweight**   BMI <5%
- **Normal weight**   BMI 5%-84%
- **Overweight**   BMI 85%-94%
- **Obese**   BMI 95%-99%
- **Morbid obesity**   BMI >99%

Fig. 1. Body mass index.

numbers are even higher among African-Americans and Hispanics, with nearly 40% of these children overweight or obese. If this trend does not change, estimates show that one-third of all children born in 2000 or later will at some point in their lives have comorbidities typically linked to excessive weight. In particular, the prevalence of metabolic syndrome has increased significantly, and more than 2 million children in the United States currently have this condition, defined by systemic hypertension, atherogenic dyslipidemia, and glucose intolerance.

OBESITY-ASTHMA LINK

A similar epidemiologic pattern has been observed for chronic respiratory diseases, particularly asthma. Four million children younger than 14 years have been diagnosed with asthma in the United States,[5] and the current global estimates of asthma prevalence range from less than 5% to more than 25%.[6] The parallel increase in obesity and asthma rates among children has led many investigators to postulate a relationship between these conditions,[7–10] although whether this relationship is causal or confounded by other factors remains a matter of debate.

Previous studies of the association between asthma and obesity have focused on 3 hypothetical mechanisms. The most simplistic theory is centered on specific nutrients, such as antioxidants and saturated fat,[7] and their role in oxidative lung damage or decreasing the lung's defenses against attacks from biological or chemical agents. The recent emphasis on the potential role of vitamin D deficiency in the pathophysiology of several chronic diseases driven by immunologic or autoimmune mechanisms, including asthma, has given new life to this idea, but the conclusions from interventional trials with high-dose vitamin D supplementation remain controversial.[11]

A second theory is centered on the mechanical effects of abdominal fat on respiratory system resistance and compliance.[8,9] Obesity reduces total lung capacity (TLC), particularly through decreasing the expiratory reserve volume and consequently the functional residual capacity. This process leads to the rapid, shallow breathing pattern that occurs close to closing volume in obese subjects. Perhaps more importantly, breathing at low TLC is associated with reduced peripheral airway diameter, and this in turn alters the bronchial smooth muscle structure and function, leading to airway hyperresponsiveness.

The third theory, which is also the most recent and probably most widely accepted, is based on the inflammatory mechanisms implicated in both conditions.[8,12] In obesity, visceral adiposity is associated with increased expression of multiple soluble mediators that amplify and propagate inflammation locally and systemically. This function involves the recruitment of inflammatory cells by chemokines, such as monocyte chemoattractant protein-1, and the direct synthesis of predominantly proinflammatory cytokines and chemokines, such as leptin, interleukin 6, tumor necrosis factor α, transforming growth factor β1, and eotaxin. The resulting perturbation of the balance between Th1 and Th2 immunomodulatory pathways, favoring the latter, has been hypothesized to be one of the mechanisms through which obesity might increase asthma risk or modify asthma phenotype.

DIABETES-ASTHMA LINK

In addition to the hypothetical relationship between obesity and asthma, strong evidence suggests that obesity is associated with the development of insulin resistance and type II diabetes.[13] In turn, diabetes and insulin resistance are associated with diminished lung function,[14–16] and some studies have also found a relationship between insulin resistance and lung function among people without diabetes, even after controlling for BMI (**Fig. 2**).

Therefore, increasing rates of pediatric asthma could result directly from peripheral tissue insulin resistance and compensatory hyperinsulinemia, which interfere with the anti-inflammatory effects of insulin while increasing bronchial reactivity through inhibition of presynaptic M2 muscarinic receptors.[17] In addition, intracellular serine/threonine kinases, such as c-Jun NH_2-terminal kinases, are activated by toll-like receptor signaling in the context of innate immunoinflammatory responses, and also inhibit insulin signaling.[18] Because of the close interdependence between inflammatory and metabolic pathways, pharmacologic ligands of the peroxisome proliferator-activated family of nuclear receptor proteins, widely used to treat hyperlipidemia and diabetes, may also treat the airway inflammation and hyperreactivity characteristic of asthma.

METABOLIC ORIGINS OF ASTHMA

Obesity has generally been thought to be the central hub from which comorbidities such as asthma, cardiovascular disease, and metabolic syndrome originate. Because of this bias, most of the studies designed to examine the interactions between childhood asthma and obesity were based on select cohorts of obese children.[19] A few years ago, the approved authors reasoned that new and important information could result from studies investigating larger, more heterogeneous samples of children stratified by body mass.[19]

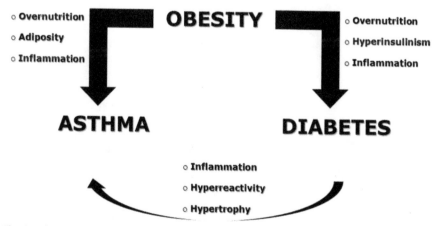

Fig. 2. Obesity-diabetes-asthma link.

A unique opportunity to fill this knowledge gap became available through collaboration with the Coronary Artery Risk Detection in Appalachian Communities (CARDIAC) Project, a federally and state-funded, community-based cardiovascular risk detection program offered to all children enrolled in kindergarten and second and fifth grades in West Virginia.[20,21] Every year, this project screens tens of thousands of children for BMI. The screening staff also explores the base of the child's neck and axilla for evidence of acanthosis nigricans (**Fig. 3**), a hyperpigmented skin rash associated with insulin resistance and hyperinsulinemia in children,[22] and a blood sample is drawn from fifth grade students only to obtain a fasting lipid profile. Before screening, parents or guardians of all participating children provide demographic and family history information by completing a questionnaire.

Analysis of almost 18,000 children enrolled during the academic year 2007–2008 provided the first conclusive evidence of the relationship between asthma and body mass in a large population of children across the entire range of weight percentile categories.[19] This analysis confirmed that asthma prevalence increases with BMI, but only when BMI reaches the obese and morbidly obese range, whereas no difference is seen in asthma prevalence among overweight versus normal weight children (**Fig. 4**). This observation suggests the existence of a threshold beyond which the metabolic derangement begins to affect airway function. Importantly, this study showed similar results in both genders, whereas a previous study in a much smaller sample suggested that body mass may affect asthma prevalence only in girls.[23]

The most important conclusion of the present study is that asthma is directly associated with elevated serum triglyceride levels and insulin resistance, regardless of BMI. This finding contributes to the mounting concern about a potentially large population of children, occasionally referred to as being "thin-fat," who are metabolically obese despite having a deceivingly normal weight. These children are at risk of being overlooked because they have a healthy appearance based on weight and adiposity, yet their metabolism is already abnormal and is predisposing them to the same cardiovascular and respiratory comorbidities typically seen in their overweight peers.

Another indirect implication of the present data is that the widely reported association between asthma and obesity may have been confounded by the coexistence of hypertriglyceridemia and insulin resistance. Children with physician-diagnosed

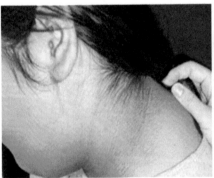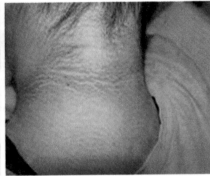

Fig. 3. Acanthosis nigricans (AN). This hyperpigmented skin rash is usually found at the base of the neck and axilla and is highly predictive of insulin resistance in adults. Although it is not as well documented in children, recent data indicate that more than 60% of children with AN also have a homeostatic model assessment index of 3 or greater. The homeostatic model assessment index is the current gold standard of insulin resistance and β-cell function based on fasting plasma glucose and insulin levels.

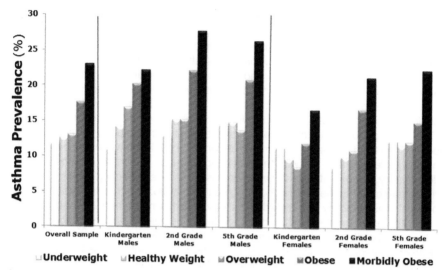

Fig. 4. Asthma prevalence based on weight category. As a general trend, asthma prevalence increases as children's BMI percentile increases. Asthma prevalence in obese and morbidly obese children is significantly higher than in children with a healthy BMI, whereas simple overweight status does not increase this risk. (*Adapted from* Cottrell L, Neal WA, Ice C, et al. Metabolic abnormalities in children with asthma. Am J Respir Crit Care Med 2011;183:443; with permission.)

asthma tend to have higher serum triglyceride levels and higher rates of insulin resistance regardless of their body mass. Thus, dyslipidemia and hyperinsulinemia, which are known silent precursors of cardiovascular disease and diabetes, may also be associated with the development of asthma, and confound its epidemiologic link to obesity.

The present findings imply a strong and direct influence of metabolic pathways on the innate and adaptive immune mechanisms involved in the pathogenesis of asthma in children, and suggest that strict monitoring and dietary/pharmacologic control of triglyceride and glucose levels starting in the first years of life may have an important role in the management of chronic asthma in children.

PRENATAL INFLUENCES

Because metabolic events have been implicated in the pathophysiology of airway inflammation and hyperreactivity, it is conceivable that early-life abnormalities in lipid and/or glucose metabolism contribute to the pathogenesis of asthma in childhood. Increasing evidence suggests that the 9 months spent in the mother's uterus and the first months after birth shape the remainder of a person's life and defines one's medical destiny.

This concept may be true also for the most common respiratory conditions, such as asthma and chronic obstructive pulmonary disease. Preliminary data from the authors' laboratory suggest that an imbalanced diet in pregnancy interferes with lung development and innervation, leading to postnatal airway hyperreactivity independent of the postnatal diet. Furthermore, the prenatal diet can also affect the development of innate and adaptive immune protection, thereby making an infant more susceptible to early-life infections, such as respiratory syncytial virus and human rhinovirus, that predispose to recurrent wheezing and asthma in childhood.

The common belief has been that nothing bad happens to the lungs until the baby is born, except in rare cases of congenital malformations or if gestation is truncated by a preterm delivery, and that the earliest manifestations of lung disease stem from noxious agents attacking the newborn lungs after birth. However, if the maternal diet affects lung development, the understanding of the pathogenesis of respiratory diseases would be completely changed. This notion would turn back the clock of respiratory developmental diseases by months and practitioners would need to start thinking about lung development and disease during pregnancy rather than at birth.

This concept could create a paradigm shift through extending the focus on prevention from the first few years after birth to also include the last few months before birth. The new paradigm is in line with the emerging evidence that many (or most) chronic inflammatory, degenerative, and even neoplastic diseases affecting adults have their origins from often-subtle events occurring during fetal life. The "fetal programming hypothesis" was originally formulated by Dr David Barker more than 2 decades ago to explain the extensively reproduced and confirmed epidemiologic evidence that low birth weight predisposes to cardiovascular disease in late adulthood.[24]

Barker's recent death leaves the legacy of this initially controversial but now widely accepted idea that common chronic illnesses such as cancer, cardiovascular disease, and diabetes do not always result from bad genes and an unhealthy adult lifestyle but rather are sometimes caused by poor intrauterine and early postnatal health. In one of his last public speeches, Barker argued, "The next generation does not have to suffer from heart disease or osteoporosis. These diseases are not mandated by the human genome. They barely existed 100 years ago. They are unnecessary diseases. We could prevent them had we the will to do so."

The authors believe the same concepts can be extended to chronic obstructive airway diseases such as asthma, which is the final product of complex interactions between genetic and environmental variables (**Fig. 5**). What makes lungs prone to develop chronic disease? Of course, genetic traits inherited from parents are important role. But also the quantity and quality of food the mother eats, the pollution in

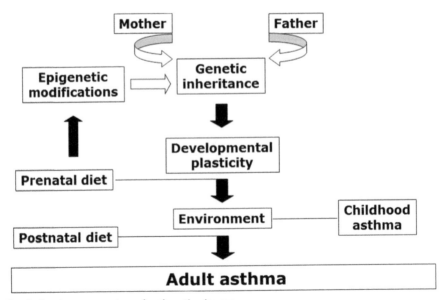

Fig. 5. Fetal programming of asthmatic airways.

the air she breathes, and the infections she sustains during gestation will play a critical role throughout a child's life, perhaps even more important than genetics. In particular, prenatal events such as intrauterine exposure to imbalanced maternal nutrition, infections, or pollutants will cause a shift in the trajectory of structural and functional airway development toward a hyperreactive phenotype. The same intrauterine exposures can affect gene expression via epigenetic modifications, such as DNA methylation and histone acetylation, and by altering the relative expression of regulatory micro-RNAs.[25]

The resulting neonatal phenotype may predispose the child to aberrant responses to common respiratory infections and airborne irritants, thereby increasing the risk of obstructive lung disease later in life. Postnatal events, such as exposure to indoor and outdoor pollutants and allergens, can further shift the equilibrium of the adult phenotype by exacerbating airway inflammation and hyperreactivity. The continuous range of possible developmental trajectories and multiple sequential events acting during development will define the severity and duration of disease.

Dr Barker believed that public health medicine was failing and that its cornerstone should be the protection of the nutrition of young women. Chronic diseases such as obesity, diabetes, and asthma are becoming epidemic, and their management in adulthood is escalating the costs of health care to proportions unsustainable for any world economy. To successfully control chronic airway diseases that so far have eluded any therapeutic strategy, it is essential to recognize that the months spent in the womb may be the most consequential of a child's life, and to identify the intrauterine and early life events that shape the development of the respiratory system to prevent or redirect dysfunctional phenotypes before they result in actual disease. Ensuring a balanced diet for all pregnant women and their newborns may one day become among the first and most important steps in this direction.

ACKNOWLEDGMENTS

The authors are very grateful to Dr W. Neil and his CARDIAC Project, without whom the research on the link between asthma, diabetes, and obesity would not have been possible. We also thank the National Heart, Lung, and Blood Institute of the National Institutes of Health for the generous support of our research over the past 15 years.

REFERENCES

1. Wojcicki JM, Heyman MB. Let's move—childhood obesity prevention from pregnancy and infancy onward. N Engl J Med 2010;362:1457–9.
2. Hammer LD, Kraemer HC, Wilson DM, et al. Standardized percentile curves of body-mass index for children and adolescents. Am J Dis Child 1991;145:259–63.
3. Ogden C, Carroll M. Prevalence of obesity among children and adolescents: United States trends 1963-1965 through 2007-2008. CDC National Center for Health Statistics. June 2010. Available at: www.cdc.gov.
4. Wojcicki JM, Heyman MB. Let's move: childhood obesity prevention from pregnancy and infancy onward. N Engl J Med 2010;362:1457–9.
5. Global surveillance, prevention and control of chronic respiratory diseases: a comprehensive approach. Geneva (Switzerland): World Health Organization; 2007.
6. Worldwide variation in prevalence of symptoms of asthma, allergic rhinoconjunctivitis, and atopic eczema: ISAAC. The International Study of Asthma and Allergies in Childhood (ISAAC) Steering Committee. Lancet 1998;351:1225–32.
7. Asher MI, Keil U, Anderson HR, et al. International Study of Asthma and Allergies in Childhood (ISAAC): rationale and methods. Eur Respir J 1995;8:483–91.

8. Beuther DA, Weiss ST, Sutherland ER. Obesity and asthma. Am J Respir Crit Care Med 2006;174:112–9.

9. Chinn S. Obesity and asthma: evidence for and against a causal relation. J Asthma 2003;40:1–16.

10. Rodriguez MA, Winkleby MA, Ahn D, et al. Identification of population subgroups of children and adolescents with high asthma prevalence: findings from the Third National Health and Nutrition Examination Survey. Arch Pediatr Adolesc Med 2002;156:269–75.

11. Gupta A, Bush A, Hawrylowicz C, et al. Vitamin D and asthma in children. Paediatr Respir Rev 2012;13:236–43.

12. Weiss ST, Shore S. Obesity and asthma: directions for research. Am J Respir Crit Care Med 2004;169:963–8.

13. Goran MI, Ball GD, Cruz ML. Obesity and risk of type 2 diabetes and cardiovascular disease in children and adolescents. J Clin Endocrinol Metab 2003;88:1417–27.

14. Engstrom G, Hedblad B, Nilsson P, et al. Lung function, insulin resistance and incidence of cardiovascular disease: a longitudinal cohort study. J Intern Med 2003;253:574–81.

15. Lawlor DA, Ebrahim S, Smith GD. Associations of measures of lung function with insulin resistance and type 2 diabetes: findings from the British Women's Heart and Health Study. Diabetologia 2004;47:195–203.

16. McKeever TM, Weston PJ, Hubbard R, et al. Lung function and glucose metabolism: an analysis of data from the Third National Health and Nutrition Examination Survey. Am J Epidemiol 2005;161:546–56.

17. Al-Shawwa BA, Al-Huniti NH, DeMattia L, et al. Asthma and insulin resistance in morbidly obese children and adolescents. J Asthma 2007;44:469–73.

18. Wellen KE, Hotamisligil GS. Inflammation, stress, and diabetes. J Clin Invest 2005;115:1111–9.

19. Cottrell L, Neal WA, Ice C, et al. Metabolic abnormalities in children with asthma. Am J Respir Crit Care Med 2011;183:441–8.

20. Demerath E, Muratova V, Spangler E, et al. School-based obesity screening in rural Appalachia. Prev Med 2003;37:553–60.

21. Neal WA, Demerath E, Gonzales E, et al. Coronary Artery Risk Detection in Appalachian Communities (CARDIAC): preliminary findings. WV Med J 2001;97:102–5.

22. Hud JA Jr, Cohen JB, Wagner JM, et al. Prevalence and significance of acanthosis nigricans in an adult obese population. Arch Dermatol 1992;128:941–4.

23. Castro-Rodríguez JA, Holberg CJ, Morgan WJ, et al. Increased incidence of asthmalike symptoms in girls who become overweight or obese during the school years. Am J Respir Crit Care Med 2001 May;163:1344–9.

24. Barker DJP. Fetal origins of coronary heart disease. Br Med J 1995;311:171–4.

25. Ruchat SM, Hivert MF, Bouchard L. Epigenetic programming of obesity and diabetes by in utero exposure to gestational diabetes mellitus. Nutr Rev 2013;71 Suppl 1:S88–94.

Obesity, Metabolic Syndrome, and Airway Disease: A Bioenergetic Problem?

Anurag Agrawal, MD, PhD, FCCP[a],*, Y.S. Prakash, MD, PhD[b,c],*

KEYWORDS

- Mitochondria • Asthma • Bioenergetics • Reactive oxygen species
- Metabolic syndrome • Arginine • Statin • Metformin

KEY POINTS

- Mitochondrial dysfunction increases severity or risk of asthma.
- Caloric excesses and reduced physical activity lead to insulin resistance, obesity, and the metabolic syndrome through abnormal mitochondrial bioenergetics.
- Caloric restriction and aerobic exercise promote mitochondrial biogenesis and improve bioenergetics. Metformin treatment recapitulates some of the effects of caloric restriction.
- Mitochondrial-targeted antioxidants like coenzyme Q10 and MitoQ may be beneficial in severe asthma.

INTRODUCTION

Asthma and obesity are twin epidemics in the developed world that are becoming increasingly prevalent globally.[1–3] Not only are obese people at increased risk of asthma, but also asthma in obese individuals does not respond as well to conventional anti-inflammatory therapy, suggesting novel pathogenic mechanisms that contribute to both asthma and obesity—two seemingly disparate diseases.[4] Such mechanisms likely relate to processes that contribute to induction or maintenance of obesity or to consequences of obesity itself.[5,6] Mitochondrial dysfunction is one such process. Here we review our current understanding of how dietary and lifestyle factors lead to changes in mitochondrial metabolism and cellular bioenergetics, inducing various components of the cardiometabolic syndrome as well as airway disease. We provide

[a] Molecular Immunogenetics Laboratory and Centre of Excellence for Translational Research in Asthma & Lung Disease, CSIR-Institute of Genomics and Integrative Biology, Mall Road, Delhi 110007, India; [b] Department of Anesthesiology, Mayo Clinic, Rochester, MN 55905, USA; [c] Department of Physiology and Biomedical Engineering, Mayo Clinic, Rochester, MN 55905, USA
* Corresponding authors. #615, CSIR Institute of Genomics and Integrative Biology, Mall Road, Delhi University, Delhi 110007, India
E-mail addresses: a.agrawal@igib.in; prakash.ys@mayo.edu

Immunol Allergy Clin N Am 34 (2014) 785–796
http://dx.doi.org/10.1016/j.iac.2014.07.004
0889-8561/14/$ – see front matter © 2014 Elsevier Inc. All rights reserved.

an overview of potential mitochondria-targeted therapies and discuss the emerging use of mesenchymal stem cells as mitochondrial donors in alleviating disease.[7]

BACKGROUND

Optimal cellular bioenergetic function is the key to health.[8] It is, therefore, not surprising that bioenergetic dysfunction is seen in multiple diseases.[9–13] Normally, energy demand of most cells is met through efficient oxidative phosphorylation reactions that occur in mitochondria.[8] A substantial reserve exists in terms of mitochondrial capacity and optimal concentrations of metabolic substrates such as glucose, permitting a matching of bioenergetic supply to demand. Conversely, inadequate numbers of mitochondria, degradation of mitochondrial function, or dysregulated substrate transport are all associated with a bioenergetic failure that can occur in disease. What is less clear is whether mitochondrial dysfunction is a trigger for or a consequence of disease. Recently, there is increasing recognition that bioenergetic failure is not just an outcome of disease, (ie, driven by earlier or more upstream mechanisms) but rather a common pathogenesis thread that links a wide range of comorbidities that occur in multifactorial diseases such as obesity, metabolic syndrome, and asthma.[9,14–16] In this review, we focus on our current understanding of bioenergetic changes in obesity, insulin resistance, and asthma, highlighting a functional basis for the intertwined epidemiology. A brief overview of normal mitochondrial metabolism follows, to provide context for disease-associated changes described subsequently.

PHYSIOLOGY

Cellular bioenergetics takes place largely within the mitochondria, which are semiautonomous organelles thought to have originated from endosymbiotic relationships between ancient eukaryotic cells and proteobacteria.[8,9] Mitochondria release energy from substrates processed through the tricarboxylic acid cycle and electron transport chain (ETC), such that carbon-hydrogen bonds are oxidized to carbon dioxide and water; the liberated energy is captured in the high-energy phosphate bond of adenosinetriphosphate (ATP). The interconversion of chemical energy is by nature an inefficient process, and tight coupling between the reactions is necessary to minimize leakage. During the necessary oxygen-dependent ATP production in the ETC, there is some electron leak, leading to the generation of reactive oxygen species (ROS) as a natural byproduct. ROS, such as superoxide and hydrogen peroxide, are highly reactive molecules that are mutagenic. Although low levels of mitochondrial ROS (mtROS) can serve physiologic functions, such as signaling, excessive levels from more leaky mitochondria can be detrimental by damaging mitochondrial DNA (mtDNA) and critical oxidative phosphorylation proteins and oxidizing the lipid membrane. Not only can they cause damage within the mitochondria, thereby setting up a spiraling decline of mitochondrial function, but can adversely impact other organelles, eventually triggering apoptosis.[8,17,18] Multiple counterregulatory mechanisms are therefore in place to monitor mitochondrial quality, degrade or disrupt poorly functioning mitochondria, maintain mitochondrial networks, and form new mitochondria as demand increases.

Mitochondrial function is also coupled to bioenergetic demand.[19] ATP, the energy currency, is exported out of mitochondria and circulated within the cell, where energy can be released by controlled hydrolysis of the phosphate bonds, forming diphosphates and monophosphates (adenosine monophosphate [AMP]). Cellular energy reserve and nutrient status is monitored through well-orchestrated machinery, including AMP-sensitive protein kinase and NAD^+-dependent deacetylase SIRT1, which regulates glucose uptake, autophagy, and mitochondrial biogenesis.[19,20]

Further, the mitochondrion is intimately coupled to overall cellular physiology via the mitochondria-associated endoplasmic reticulum membrane, which regulates lipid and sterol metabolism and calcium signaling. As a result, mitochondria exhibit plasticity (ie, rapid alteration of their numbers and characteristics in response to metabolic fluctuations for meeting cellular needs).[19,21,22] Diet, exercise, insulin, and drugs strongly shape this plastic behavior and consequently mitochondrial health.

Fig. 1 illustrates the central role of mitochondria in energy metabolism. High mitochondrial reserve, low baseline ROS production, low burden of mtDNA damage, balanced cellular demand and nutrient supply, and high levels of endogenous ROS scavengers characterize health. It is notable that the inverse occurs during natural aging, obesity, and inflammatory disease (**Fig. 2**).

PATHOPHYSIOLOGY
Mitochondrial Dysfunction and Metabolic Syndrome

Caloric excess and reduced physical activity are increasingly prevalent aspects of the modern lifestyle. Surplus nutrient supply overloads mitochondria,[23] leading to overproduction of ROS and accumulation of incompletely oxidized substrates. Damage from these ROS can reduce mitochondrial integrity, triggering their clearance, and can also activate stress pathways that reduce insulin sensitivity and thereby limit nutrient uptake.[24,25] Chronic nutrient oversupply leads to oxidative stress, mitochondrial loss, and reduced maximal oxygen consumption. This is exacerbated by physical inactivity, as adaptive mechanisms for increasing mitochondrial activity or mitochondrial biogenesis are strongly related to aerobic exercise.[20] Together, this appears to be the foundation of insulin resistance, and numerous studies in humans and animal models have confirmed that insulin resistance is associated with reduced mitochondrial mass or oxidative function in insulin-sensitive tissues. This sets off a vicious

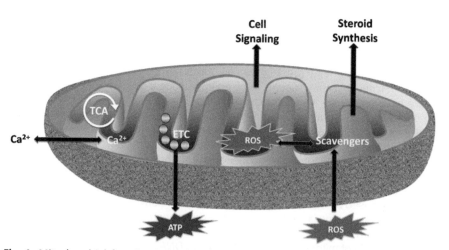

Fig. 1. Mitochondrial function in health. Mitochondria are the powerhouses of cells. The tricarboxylic/citric acid cycle (TCA) and ETC work in conjunction with glycolysis and fatty acid oxidation to extract the energy stored in carbon-hydrogen bonds and store it in ATP, which is the energy currency of the cell. ROS are generated during flow of electrons across ETC, which are scavenged by local antioxidants. A low level of ROS is important in cell signaling, and, other than ATP production, mitochondria also participate in calcium regulation and steroid synthesis.

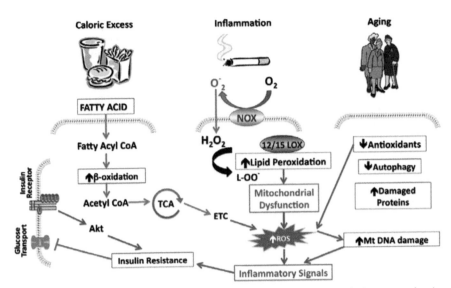

Fig. 2. Mitochondrial dysfunction is a common point of convergence during normal aging or pathologic stress. Activation of NADPH oxidase (NOX) or 12/15 lipoxygenase (LOX) is an important trigger for lipid peroxidation during inflammatory states. Increased ROS generation caused by nutrient excess or accumulation of damage with age can lead to similar endpoints.

feed-forward loop, as insulin action is important in maintaining mitochondrial metabolism and biogenesis. Because fatty acid oxidation for energy can only happen in mitochondria, fats are not adequately metabolized, leading to intracellular accumulation and increased circulating lipids. Hyperinsulinemia is the primary compensatory response to insulin resistance in the principal glucose, utilizing organs such as liver and skeletal muscle, creating β cell stress and eventually secretory deficiency. Together this forms the basis for the triad of obesity, dyslipidemia, and hyperglycemia, namely the metabolic syndrome.

Metabolic syndrome, especially obesity, represents a strong risk factor for asthma.[3,6] Hyperinsulinemia seems to be an independent risk factor in some studies, and we have previously reviewed how hyperinsulinemia may lead to changes in the lung characteristic of asthma via growth factor–like effects and increased PI3/Akt signaling.[26] Recently, a vagally mediated bronchoconstrictor effect of hyperinsulinemia has also been described.[27] These associations form the basis of exploring whether and how mitochondrial mechanisms important in metabolic syndrome can also contribute to asthma.

In the cascade of events described previously, the key initiator is mitochondrial dysfunction caused by caloric excesses and physical inactivity. So far, there is no clear evidence that this finding is related to mitochondrial genome variations, although some mtDNA polymorphisms are associated with metabolic syndrome components.[28] Although the ratio of mitochondrial DNA to nuclear DNA is markedly reduced in metabolic syndrome, it is not associated with any major genomic deletions and most likely simply represents increased damage, accelerated clearance, and, importantly, reduced mitochondrial biogenesis.[29,30] The resultant mitochondrial dysfunction, especially in key insulin-sensitive tissues like liver and muscle, potentiates hyperinsulinemia and obesity, which increase asthma risk through several pathways as discussed in this special issue and elsewhere.[3,5,6] Restricting calories and maintaining physically active lifestyles protect against such mitochondrial dysfunction, lead to weight loss, and are shown to improve asthma.[4] However, beyond this indirect link among metabolic syndrome, mitochondrial dysfunction, and asthma that is mediated by obesity and insulin resistance, there is also a much more direct link within the lung.

Mitochondrial Dysfunction and Asthma

As far back as 1985, it had been described that human bronchial epithelial cells of asthmatics showed swollen mitochondria.[31] Mabalirajan and colleagues[32,33] dissected this further in experimental mouse models of allergic airway inflammation and found this to be an integral part of the asthma phenotype. Key inflammatory cytokines associated with asthma such as interleukin-4 and inaterleukin-13 are found to induce mitochondrial dysfunction via upregulation of the oxidized linoleic acid metabolite, 13-S-HODE.[33–35] Also, allergic airway inflammation is associated with increase in asymmetric dimethyl arginine (ADMA), an endogenous methyl-arginine that uncouples nitric oxide synthase, leading to ROS formation and mitochondrial dysfunction.[36,37] Interestingly, ADMA is also increased in obesity because of increased protein turnover.[6] A causal role for mitochondrial dysfunction was further suggested by studies in mice with a genetic deficiency of mitochondrial ubiquinol-cytochrome C-reductase core II protein in the airway epithelium.[38] These mice, which have airway mitochondrial dysfunction, exhibited much greater inflammation and airway remodeling than normal mice during allergen sensitization and challenge.[38] In other work, treatment of mice with low-dose inhaled rotenone, an ETC blocker, led to features of airway remodeling and hyperresponsiveness.[7] Importantly, both mice treated with rotenone and those with allergic airway inflammation, show marked attenuation of asthmatic features if mitochondrial function is restored (see later discussion).

Currently, there is limited human evidence for a causal role of mitochondrial dysfunction in asthma. However, human genetic studies of asthma are suggestive of a mitochondrial component.[39] Although there are no consistent reports of mitochondrial mutations in asthma, vertical transmission from mothers has been reported along with some genetic associations.[40–42] Mutations in genes encoding mitochondrial tRNAs and the ATP synthase mitochondrial F1 complex assembly factor 1 gene have been associated with childhood asthma. This evidence together with experimental observations, suggest a direct role of mitochondrial dysfunction in asthma pathogenesis. What is less clear is which aspects of mitochondrial function or dysfunction contribute to human asthma phenotype, particularly along the spectrum of mild through severe asthma. It also remains unclear whether mitochondria contribute to the sensitivity or resistance of asthmatic airways to existing therapies such as corticosteroids. It is well known that mitochondria have a complex morphology because of highly regulated fission and fusion and normally form an intricate tuboloreticular branched network.[14,43] It is now also apparent that this structure has multiple and far-reaching implications, including protecting mitochondrial stability, respiratory functions, cell fate determination, and adaptation to cellular stress. Mitochondrial fragmentation and other morphologic changes occur during allergic asthma, cigarette smoke exposure, or diet-induced obesity.[14,44] These issues are not fully reversed by anti-inflammatory therapy and may contribute to progressive disease.

Mitochondrial Dysfunction and Chronic Obstructive Pulmonary Disease

Cigarette smoking and second-hand exposure increase the risk or severity of asthma and chronic obstructive pulmonary disease (COPD). Short-term as well as longer exposure to cigarette smoke are found to induce mitochondrial dysfunction.[45,46] This is accompanied by increased mitochondrial network fragmentation and ROS generation, which can be perpetuated by cell signaling pathways such as ERK, PI3/Akt, PKC and transcriptional regulation by NFκB and Nrf2.[14] This finding represents an important intersection between asthma and COPD, as airway smooth muscle (ASM) cells from asthmatics show such fragmentation and ROS generation at baseline, which is further enhanced by cigarette smoke.[14] Oxidative stress is well known as an important part of asthma and COPD pathogenesis, and there is well-known mitochondrial pathology in skeletal muscle of COPD patients.[9,47] It seems likely, therefore, that cigarette smoke–induced mitochondrial dysfunction potentiates oxidative stress in the lung, contributing to cell senescence and apoptosis. These issues represent a form of accelerated aging of the lung, which has been recently implicated in the genesis of COPD.[48–50]

TREATMENT

Currently, there is no specific approved therapy for mitochondrial dysfunction or separate treatment guidelines for obese patients with asthma. There is, however, increasing recognition that such obese-asthma is clinically different and may not respond fully to convention anti-inflammatory therapy (see review by Sherry Farzan elsewhere in this issue). The accompanying review by Nijra Lugogo in this issue, describes the role of weight loss in the management of asthma and evaluates the evidence for bariatric surgery in obese-asthma. Here we briefly focus on therapies that are associated with improvement in mitochondrial function that are shown to have potential benefit in metabolic syndrome and asthma (**Fig. 3**).

Lifestyle modification and weight loss should be first-line recommendations in obese-asthma, because they have general health benefits. Exercise and caloric restriction are found to enhance natural antioxidant scavengers, reduce mtROS, promote mitochondrial biogenesis, and slow aging.[20,51,52] However, it is also possible

Therapies associated with improvement in mitochondrial function

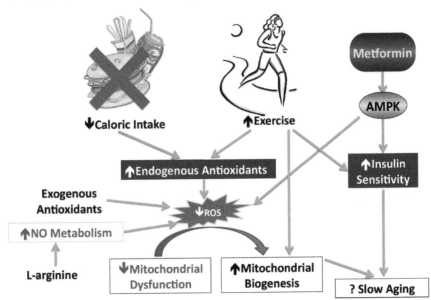

Fig. 3. Reversing bioenergetic failure in obesity and asthma.

that caloric restriction may not be acceptable to the patient, and exercise capacity may be impaired by the combination of asthma and obesity. Accordingly, although diet and lifestyle changes can have substantial beneficial effects in the context of asthma, more directed therapies are needed.

One approach toward chemically mimicking caloric restriction is to administer metformin, which via its actions on AMP-sensitive protein kinase, restores insulin sensitivity and promotes mitochondrial metabolism.[53] Metformin is already the treatment of choice for diabetes and is being considered for use in obese nondiabetics.[54] In mice with high-fat, diet-induced obesity, metformin attenuates allergen-induced eosinophilic inflammation.[55] Metformin-treated animals behaved similarly to lean controls, hastening the resolution of inflammation. Antiasthma effects of metformin were also noted in other allergen models of asthma[56] but not in genetically obese mice with intrinsic airway hyperresponsiveness or ozone-induced inflammation.[57] This finding suggests that the beneficial effects of metformin are through common metabolic processes between allergic asthma and dietary obesity, although these remain to be fully characterized.

Nitric oxide metabolism is impaired in obesity and metabolic syndrome because of increased methyl-arginines such as ADMA and reduced L-arginine bioavailability. These have also been strongly implicated in mitochondrial dysfunction and asthma. Previously we found that supplementation of L-arginine not only benefits cardiovascular aspects of the metabolic syndrome but also attenuates mitochondrial dysfunction and asthma features in experimental models.[36,58] Similar effects on nitric oxide metabolism and asthma were obtained by inhibition of L-arginine degradation by arginase[59] or by statin-mediated restoration of eNOS levels and degrading of ADMA.[60] Even metformin has important effects of nitric oxide metabolism, suggesting that this may be a critical common interface between obesity and asthma. These drugs are now in clinical trial for asthma, and the review elsewhere in this issue by Nicholas Kenyon, on novel therapeutic strategies for obese-asthma, provides more detail.

Exogenous antioxidants to scavenge ROS, inhibitors of 12/15 lipoxygenase (baicalein and esculetin) to reduce mitotoxicity, and sirtuin activators such as resveratrol to stimulate mitochondrial biogenesis, have all been found to attenuate experimental asthma.[43,61–64] Although these pathways are also implicated in obesity and metabolic syndrome, any benefits of these strategies in obese-asthma remain to be ascertained.

Mitochondria-targeted antioxidants are also of potential benefit. Coenzyme Q10 (CoQ10), also known as ubiquinone, is a component of the ETC and can, therefore, exist in both fully oxidized and reduced states, making it a powerful mitochondria-targeted antioxidant.[65] In a small study of 56 asthmatics, Gazdik and colleagues[66] reported reduction of CoQ10 in plasma and whole blood. In a subsequent open-label crossover study of 41 steroid-dependent asthma patients, they found that supplementation with a daily antioxidant cocktail, consisting of CoQ10 (120 mg) + 400 mg α-tocopherol + 250 mg vitamin C, was associated with a reduction in steroid usage.[67] Because glucocorticoids can induce mitochondrial dysfunction and are relatively ineffective in obese-asthma, this is potentially important. CoQ supplementation is also variably found to be beneficial in cardiac components of the metabolic syndrome.[68] However, supplementation with other exogenous antioxidants like α-tocopherol and vitamin C have not been successful, and there are conflicting reports including interference with mitochondrial signaling and biogenesis.[69] Thus, mitochondria-targeted antioxidants such as CoQ10 and its modified forms (MitoQ) merit further investigation in the treatment of obese-asthma.[70]

One limitation of any mitochondrial-targeted therapy in asthma is that mitochondrial numbers and dysfunction in different cell types may have different implications and may even be a double-edged sword.[9,14,71] For example, ROS produced during fatty acid oxidation in mitochondria suppress the inflammatory Th17 lymphocyte polarization, and dominant fatty acid metabolism promotes formation of regulatory T cells that have important anti-inflammatory function.[71] Thus, normal mitochondrial ROS generation can be beneficial, and antioxidant therapy may not always be helpful. However, airway epithelial cells from allergically inflamed lungs show increased ROS, mitochondrial dysfunction, and a reduction in mitochondrial biogenesis.[7] The ASM shows increased mitochondrial fission, dysfunctional mitochondrial network formation, and increased ROS, although the biogenesis may be increased.[7,14] Together, these promote the aberrant fibrotic and hypercontractile pathology of asthma that is characterized by epithelial injury but ASM and fibroblast proliferation. An additional layer of cell-type specific targeting, either through delivery routes and carriers or through novel biologicals, may be required to specifically target mitochondrial function.

SUMMARY AND FUTURE DIRECTIONS

Both obesity and asthma share common metabolic derangements that intersect at the level of mitochondrial function. It is likely that the mitochondrial dysfunction of insulin resistance or obesity increases asthma incidence or severity. Conversely, asthma-associated mitochondrial dysfunction may lead to systemic metabolic changes that promote insulin resistance and obesity.[72] Several clinical trials are in progress for evaluation of metabolic drugs like metformin, statins, and L-arginine in asthma, and the results are awaited. Mitochondrial-targeted antioxidants like CoQ10 and MitoQ also show promise. Until recently there were no strategies for replenishing healthy mitochondria and restoring normal bioenergetics by exogenous donation. However, recent

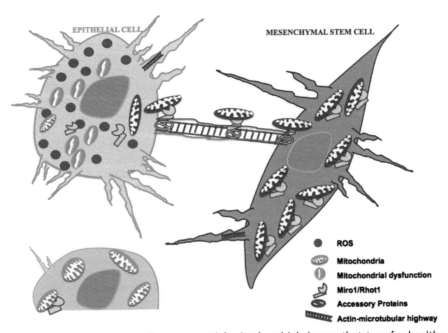

Fig. 4. Mesenchymal stem cells are potential mitochondrial donors that transfer healthy mitochondria via intercellular nanotubes to stressed epithelial cells. In experimental models, this has been associated with antiasthma effects.

work from Jahar Bhattacharya's laboratory[73] and the Agrawal lab[7] shows that exogenous mesenchymal stem cells (MSC) can donate mitochondria to lung epithelium, restoring bioenergetic function and attenuating inflammation and injury. This transfer seems to be regulated by Miro1, a GTPase, and MSC that overexpress Miro1 show amplification of mitochondrial donation as well as increased therapeutic efficacy in reversing experimental asthma.[7] This is being explored further in models of diet-induced obesity, metabolic syndrome, and asthma and represents an entirely new direction for the future (**Fig. 4**).

ACKNOWLEDGMENTS

This work was supported by the Lady Tata Memorial Trust (GAP63) and Council of Scientific and Industrial Research grant MLP5502 (A. Agrawal) and National Institutes of Health Grants HL088029 and HL056470 (Y.S. Prakash). The authors thank Shravani Mukherjee and Rohit Vashisht for their help.

REFERENCES

1. Kent BD, Lane SJ. Twin epidemics: asthma and obesity. Int Arch Allergy Immunol 2012;157:213–4.
2. Brisbon N, Plumb J, Brawer R, et al. The asthma and obesity epidemics: the role played by the built environment–a public health perspective. J Allergy Clin Immunol 2005;115:1024–8.
3. Beuther DA. Recent insight into obesity and asthma. Curr Opin Pulm Med 2010; 16:64–70.
4. Farzan S. The asthma phenotype in the obese: distinct or otherwise? J Allergy (Cairo) 2013;2013:602908.
5. Agrawal A, Sood A, Linneberg A, et al. Mechanistic understanding of the effect of obesity on asthma and allergy. J Allergy (Cairo) 2013;2013:598904.
6. Agrawal A, Mabalirajan U, Ahmad T, et al. Emerging interface between metabolic syndrome and asthma. Am J Respir Cell Mol Biol 2011;44(3):270–5.
7. Ahmad T, Mukherjee S, Pattnaik B, et al. Miro1 regulates intercellular mitochondrial transport & enhances mesenchymal stem cell rescue efficacy. EMBO J 2014;33(9):994–1010.
8. Hill BG, Benavides GA, Lancaster JR Jr, et al. Integration of cellular bioenergetics with mitochondrial quality control and autophagy. Biol Chem 2012;393: 1485–512.
9. Aravamudan B, Thompson MA, Pabelick CM, et al. Mitochondria in lung diseases. Expert Rev Respir Med 2013;7:631–46.
10. Lee HK, Park KS, Cho YM, et al. Mitochondria-based model for fetal origin of adult disease and insulin resistance. Ann N Y Acad Sci 2005;1042:1–18.
11. Irving BA, Nair KS. Aging and diabetes: mitochondrial dysfunction. Curr Diab Rep 2007;7:249–51.
12. Vernochet C, Kahn CR. Mitochondria, obesity and aging. Aging (Albany NY) 2012;4:859–60.
13. Martin SD, McGee SL. The role of mitochondria in the aetiology of insulin resistance and type 2 diabetes. Biochim Biophys Acta 2014;1840:1303–12.
14. Aravamudan B, Kiel A, Freeman M, et al. Cigarette smoke-induced mitochondrial fragmentation and dysfunction in human airway smooth muscle. Am J Physiol Lung Cell Mol Physiol 2014;306(9):L840–54.
15. Naviaux RK. Metabolic features of the cell danger response. Mitochondrion 2013;16:7–17.

16. Mabalirajan U, Ghosh B. Mitochondrial dysfunction in metabolic syndrome and asthma. J Allergy (Cairo) 2013;2013:340476.
17. Farid S, Mirshafiey A, Razavi A. Siglec-8 and Siglec-F, the new therapeutic targets in asthma. Immunopharmacol Immunotoxicol 2012;34:721–6.
18. Roscioli E, Hamon R, Ruffin RE, et al. Cellular inhibitor of apoptosis-2 is a critical regulator of apoptosis in airway epithelial cells treated with asthma-related inflammatory cytokines. Physiol Rep 2013;1:e00123.
19. Cheng Z, Ristow M. Mitochondria and metabolic homeostasis. Antioxid Redox Signal 2013;19:240–2.
20. Lanza IR, Short DK, Short KR, et al. Endurance exercise as a countermeasure for aging. Diabetes 2008;57:2933–42.
21. Jelenik T, Roden M. Mitochondrial plasticity in obesity and diabetes mellitus. Antioxid Redox Signal 2013;19:258–68.
22. Martin-Montalvo A, de Cabo R. Mitochondrial metabolic reprogramming induced by calorie restriction. Antioxid Redox Signal 2013;19:310–20.
23. Cheng Z, Almeida FA. Mitochondrial alteration in type 2 diabetes and obesity: an epigenetic link. Cell Cycle 2014;13:890–7.
24. Hancock CR, Han DH, Chen M, et al. High-fat diets cause insulin resistance despite an increase in muscle mitochondria. Proc Natl Acad Sci U S A 2008; 105:7815–20.
25. Watt MJ, Hevener AL. Fluxing the mitochondria to insulin resistance. Cell Metab 2008;7:5–6.
26. Singh S, Prakash YS, Linneberg A, et al. Insulin and the lung: connecting asthma and metabolic syndrome. J Allergy (Cairo) 2013;2013:627384.
27. Nie Z, Jacoby DB, Fryer AD. Hyperinsulinemia potentiates airway responsiveness to parasympathetic nerve stimulation in obese rats. Am J Respir Cell Mol Biol 2014;51(2):251–61.
28. Palmieri VO, De Rasmo D, Signorile A, et al. T16189C mitochondrial DNA variant is associated with metabolic syndrome in Caucasian subjects. Nutrition 2011; 27:773–7.
29. Gemma C, Sookoian S, Dieuzeide G, et al. Methylation of TFAM gene promoter in peripheral white blood cells is associated with insulin resistance in adolescents. Mol Genet Metab 2010;100:83–7.
30. Gianotti TF, Sookoian S, Dieuzeide G, et al. A decreased mitochondrial DNA content is related to insulin resistance in adolescents. Obesity (Silver Spring) 2008;16:1591–5.
31. Konradova V, Copova C, Sukova B, et al. Ultrastructure of the bronchial epithelium in three children with asthma. Pediatr Pulmonol 1985;1:182–7.
32. Mabalirajan U, Dinda AK, Kumar S, et al. Mitochondrial structural changes and dysfunction are associated with experimental allergic asthma. J Immunol 2008; 181:3540–8.
33. Mabalirajan U, Rehman R, Ahmad T, et al. 12/15-lipoxygenase expressed in non-epithelial cells causes airway epithelial injury in asthma. Sci Rep 2013;3:1540.
34. Rehman R, Bhat YA, Panda L, et al. TRPV1 inhibition attenuates IL-13 mediated asthma features in mice by reducing airway epithelial injury. Int Immunopharmacol 2013;15:597–605.
35. Mabalirajan U, Rehman R, Ahmad T, et al. Linoleic acid metabolite drives severe asthma by causing airway epithelial injury. Sci Rep 2013;3:1349.
36. Mabalirajan U, Ahmad T, Leishangthem GD, et al. L-arginine reduces mitochondrial dysfunction and airway injury in murine allergic airway inflammation. Int Immunopharmacol 2010;10:1514–9.

37. Ahmad T, Mabalirajan U, Ghosh B, et al. Altered asymmetric dimethyl arginine metabolism in allergically inflamed mouse lungs. Am J Respir Cell Mol Biol 2010;42:3–8.
38. Aguilera-Aguirre L, Bacsi A, Saavedra-Molina A, et al. Mitochondrial dysfunction increases allergic airway inflammation. J Immunol 2009;183:5379–87.
39. Flaquer A, Heinzmann A, Rospleszcz S, et al. Association study of mitochondrial genetic polymorphisms in asthmatic children. Mitochondrion 2014;14: 49–53.
40. Litonjua AA, Carey VJ, Burge HA, et al. Parental history and the risk for childhood asthma. Does mother confer more risk than father? Am J Respir Crit Care Med 1998;158:176–81.
41. Schauberger EM, Ewart SL, Arshad SH, et al. Identification of ATPAF1 as a novel candidate gene for asthma in children. J Allergy Clin Immunol 2011;128: 753–60.e11.
42. Zifa E, Daniil Z, Skoumi E, et al. Mitochondrial genetic background plays a role in increasing risk to asthma. Mol Biol Rep 2012;39:4697–708.
43. Ahmad T, Aggarwal K, Pattnaik B, et al. Computational classification of mitochondrial shapes reflects stress and redox state. Cell Death Dis 2013;4:e461.
44. Leishangthem GD, Mabalirajan U, Singh VP, et al. Ultrastructural changes of airway in murine models of allergy and diet-induced metabolic syndrome. ISRN Allergy 2013;2013:261297.
45. Agarwal AR, Yin F, Cadenas E. Short-term cigarette smoke exposure leads to metabolic alterations in lung alveolar cells. Am J Respir Cell Mol Biol 2014; 51(2):284–93.
46. Hoffmann RF, Zarrintan S, Brandenburg SM, et al. Prolonged cigarette smoke exposure alters mitochondrial structure and function in airway epithelial cells. Respir Res 2013;14:97.
47. Puente-Maestu L, Perez-Parra J, Godoy R, et al. Abnormal transition pore kinetics and cytochrome C release in muscle mitochondria of patients with chronic obstructive pulmonary disease. Am J Respir Cell Mol Biol 2009;40: 746–50.
48. Ito K, Colley T, Mercado N. Geroprotectors as a novel therapeutic strategy for COPD, an accelerating aging disease. Int J Chron Obstruct Pulmon Dis 2012; 7:641–52.
49. Ito K, Barnes PJ. COPD as a disease of accelerated lung aging. Chest 2009; 135:173–80.
50. MacNee W. Accelerated lung aging: a novel pathogenic mechanism of chronic obstructive pulmonary disease (COPD). Biochem Soc Trans 2009;37:819–23.
51. Hoeks J, Schrauwen P. Muscle mitochondria and insulin resistance: a human perspective. Trends Endocrinol Metab 2012;23:444–50.
52. Lanza IR, Nair KS. Muscle mitochondrial changes with aging and exercise. Am J Clin Nutr 2009;89:467S–71S.
53. Martin-Montalvo A, Mercken EM, Mitchell SJ, et al. Metformin improves healthspan and lifespan in mice. Nat Commun 2013;4:2192.
54. Golay A. Metformin and body weight. Int J Obes (Lond) 2008;32:61–72.
55. Calixto MC, Lintomen L, Andre DM, et al. Metformin attenuates the exacerbation of the allergic eosinophilic inflammation in high fat-diet-induced obesity in mice. PLoS One 2013;8:e76786.
56. Park CS, Bang BR, Kwon HS, et al. Metformin reduces airway inflammation and remodeling via activation of AMP-activated protein kinase. Biochem Pharmacol 2012;84:1660–70.

57. Shore SA, Williams ES, Zhu M. No effect of metformin on the innate airway hyperresponsiveness and increased responses to ozone observed in obese mice. J Appl Physiol (1985) 2008;105:1127–33.

58. Mabalirajan U, Ahmad T, Leishangthem GD, et al. Beneficial effects of high dose of L-arginine on airway hyperresponsiveness and airway inflammation in a murine model of asthma. J Allergy Clin Immunol 2010;125:626–35.

59. Mabalirajan U, Aich J, Agrawal A, et al. Mepacrine inhibits subepithelial fibrosis by reducing the expression of arginase and TGF-beta1 in an extended subacute mouse model of allergic asthma. Am J Physiol Lung Cell Mol Physiol 2009;297:L411–9.

60. Ahmad T, Mabalirajan U, Sharma A, et al. Simvastatin improves epithelial dysfunction and airway hyperresponsiveness: from ADMA to asthma. Am J Respir Cell Mol Biol 2010;44(4):531–9.

61. Mabalirajan U, Ahmad T, Rehman R, et al. Baicalein reduces airway injury in allergen and IL-13 induced airway inflammation. PLoS One 2013;8:e62916.

62. Aich J, Mabalirajan U, Ahmad T, et al. Resveratrol attenuates experimental allergic asthma in mice by restoring inositol polyphosphate 4 phosphatase (INPP4A). Int Immunopharmacol 2012;14:438–43.

63. Mabalirajan U, Aich J, Leishangthem GD, et al. Effects of vitamin E on mitochondrial dysfunction and asthma features in an experimental allergic murine model. J Appl Physiol (1985) 2009;107:1285–92.

64. Mabalirajan U, Dinda AK, Sharma SK, et al. Esculetin restores mitochondrial dysfunction and reduces allergic asthma features in experimental murine model. J Immunol 2009;183:2059–67.

65. Madmani ME, Solaiman AY, Tamr Agha K, et al. Coenzyme Q10 for heart failure. Cochrane Database Syst Rev 2013;(9):CD008684.

66. Gazdik F, Gvozdjakova A, Horvathova M, et al. Levels of coenzyme Q10 in asthmatics. Bratisl Lek Listy 2002;103:353–6.

67. Gvozdjakova A, Kucharska J, Bartkovjakova M, et al. Coenzyme Q10 supplementation reduces corticosteroids dosage in patients with bronchial asthma. Biofactors 2005;25:235–40.

68. Littarru GP, Tiano L. Clinical aspects of coenzyme Q10: an update. Nutrition 2010;26:250–4.

69. Gomez-Cabrera MC, Domenech E, Romagnoli M, et al. Oral administration of vitamin C decreases muscle mitochondrial biogenesis and hampers training-induced adaptations in endurance performance. Am J Clin Nutr 2008;87:142–9.

70. Armstrong JS. Mitochondria-directed therapeutics. Antioxid Redox Signal 2008; 10:575–8.

71. Barbi J, Pardoll D, Pan F. Metabolic control of the Treg/Th17 axis. Immunol Rev 2013;252:52–77.

72. Cottrell L, Neal WA, Ice C, et al. Metabolic abnormalities in children with asthma. Am J Respir Crit Care Med 2011;183:441–8.

73. Islam MN, Das SR, Emin MT, et al. Mitochondrial transfer from bone-marrow-derived stromal cells to pulmonary alveoli protects against acute lung injury. Nat Med 2012;18:759–65.

Role of Weight Management in Asthma Symptoms and Control

Timothy Heacock, MD, Njira Lugogo, MD*

KEYWORDS

- Obesity • Asthma • Weight loss • Gastric bypass surgery • Asthma control

KEY POINTS

- Weight loss achieved by both dietary and surgical interventions improves asthma symptoms and control.
- There may a subset of obese patients with asthma who receive added benefits from weight loss. These patients tend to have late-onset asthma that is preceded by obesity and have decreased airway hyperresponsiveness with weight loss.
- More research is needed to determine whether the physiologic changes that occur with obesity are responsible for the improvements in asthma symptoms.
- Weight loss should be recommended to patients with poor asthma control; however, there are insufficient data to support surgical interventions for weight loss solely for the purpose of improving asthma control.

INTRODUCTION

The prevalence of obesity has increased significantly over the past several decades, with more than a third of adults in the United States now considered obese (body mass index [BMI] >30) according to a recent report from the US Centers for Disease Control and Prevention. Obesity has a known association with diabetes mellitus type 2, hypertension, and atherosclerotic heart disease. Over the past decade it has become increasingly recognized that obesity is associated with asthma, with an increased risk of developing asthma with increasing BMI in a dose-response manner.[1] In addition, overweight/obese patients with asthma have more symptoms, poor asthma control, and decreased response to conventional asthma therapies, including inhaled steroids.[2] Patients who are morbidly obese bear the greatest morbidity from asthma and the prevalence of asthma in the bariatric surgery population is as high

Conflicts of interest: Drs T. Heacock and N. Lugogo have no conflicts of interest related to the topic of this article.
Department of Pulmonary and Critical Care, Duke University Medical Center, Durham, NC 27710, USA
* Corresponding author.
E-mail address: njira.lugogo@duke.edu

as 10%.[3] Obesity has also been recognized as a risk factor for more severe and difficult-to-treat asthma, and obese patients with asthma have poor response to conventional asthma therapies including inhaled steroids, which is thought to be caused by glucocorticoid resistance.[2,4,5] Animal models and epidemiologic studies have suggested that leptin, a hormone that regulates satiety and is increased in obesity, and adiponectin, an antiinflammatory hormone that is present in decreased levels in obesity, may play a role in allergic airway inflammation and subsequently cause worsening asthma.[6,7] Proposed mechanisms for the increased risk of asthma in obesity include shallow tidal breathing caused by decreased chest wall compliance causing decreased airway smooth muscle stretch and increased hyperresponsiveness, increased incidence of gastroesophageal reflux, sleep-disordered breathing (SDB), misdiagnosis of asthma, genetic polymorphism, and effects of systemic cytokines associated with obesity on inflammation in the lungs.[8–11] There is likely a causal relationship between obesity and asthma and thus targeting weight loss in individuals who are overweight/obese with asthma is likely to lead to improved asthma control and may even cause reversal of inflammation and potentially fully resolve asthma in patients for whom obesity is the primary cause of disease.

This article discusses the effect of weight loss via dietary modifications and surgical interventions on asthma symptoms and control. It is concerned with the effect of weight loss on inflammatory mediators of asthma and the impact of alterations in inflammation on asthma.

DIETARY INTERVENTIONS IN WEIGHT MANAGEMENT

There are several observational studies that have been performed to determine the effect of changes in weight on asthma control and symptoms (**Table 1**). A study from the United Kingdom followed 151 patients with severe asthma (75% with BMI>25 and 44% with BMI>30) over a 1-year period and monitored changes in their weight. There was no correlation with changes in weight and asthma exacerbations or Asthma Control Questionnaire (ACQ) scores. However, there was a correlation between weight change and forced expiratory volume in 1 second (FEV_1) with increased FEV_1 associated with decreases in weight ($r = -0.3$; $P = .03$).[12] In a larger cohort of patients, Haselkorn and colleagues[13] evaluated patients from The Epidemiology and Natural history of Asthma: Outcomes and Treatment Regimens (TENOR) study with severe or difficult-to-treat asthma divided into 3 groups based on changes in weight over a 1-year period. The groups were divided into those patients that had greater than or equal to 2.3-kg (5-lb) weight loss, less than 2.3-kg change in weight, or greater than or equal to 2.3-kg weight gain. Those who gained weight reported poor asthma control and required a greater number of steroid bursts for asthma exacerbations. The patients who lost weight did not experience improvements in asthma control. However, this study is limited by the inclusion of nonobese individuals and the low threshold of weight loss that is likely to result in low power to detect a difference in asthma control associated with weight loss.

These observational studies indicated that obesity is associated with poorer asthma control, quality of life, and increased exposure to oral steroids. In these initial studies the effect of weight loss on lung function measures was unclear because there were contrary findings with regard to FEV_1. Based on these findings, several investigators designed studies that incorporated weight loss interventions to determine the effect of weight loss on markers of asthma control, quality of life, and lung function measures.

Stenius-Aarniala and colleagues[14] completed an unblinded randomized controlled trial of 38 obese patients with asthma assessing the effects of a 14-week weight reduction program using a low-calorie diet (1757 kJ [420 cal]) versus no intervention. The subjects in the intervention group lost 14.5% of their pretreatment weight and this weight loss was sustained at 11.3% after 1 year. In comparison, the controls lost 0.3% during the study and gained 2.2% of their pretreatment weight at 1 year. The intervention group showed improvements in FEV_1, forced vital capacity (FVC), use of rescue medication, and number of exacerbations at the conclusion of the study. The improvements in FEV_1 and FVC persisted at the 1-year follow-up visit; however, the improvement in rescue medication use was no longer significant. Although there was no improvement in health status based on the St George's Respiratory Questionnaire at the conclusion of the study, there were significant differences in scores at 6 months and a year. This study was the first to show that a nonsurgical weight loss intervention could lead to sustained improvement in lung function and health status. In a follow-up study by the same investigators, 14 subjects had significant improvements in peak expiratory flow (PEF) diurnal variation, day-to-day PEF variation, and airway resistance with similar improvements in FEV_1 and FVC.[15] Based on these findings, the investigators suggested that weight loss may improve asthma through changes in lung mechanics and decreased airway obstruction.

Johnson and colleagues[16] noted improvements in self-reported symptoms and PEF rate but not FEV_1 with an alternating-day low-calorie diet that resulted in an average of 8.5% loss of pretreatment weight. The improvements in lung function occurred within 2 weeks of initiating the diet, suggesting that changes in inflammatory mediators and other effects of changes in diet may have caused improvements in lung function even in the absence of significant weight loss. Other studies have noted similar improvements in need for rescue bronchodilator use associated with dietary modifications exclusive of weight loss. Hernandez Romero[17] showed that subjects treated with a premixed protein powder diet did not require albuterol during the study, compared with 90% of patients requiring albuterol for rescue in the group receiving a personalized meal plan. The difference in rescue medication use may be explained partially by the difference in the dietary interventions (ie, components of the two diets) or a greater decrease in BMI.

If asthma is a consequence of systemic changes associated with diet and not obesity alone, then dietary changes may mitigate inflammation via alteration of systemic cytokines or changes in the microbiome with downstream alteration of immune responses. This alteration would be a plausible explanation for why asthma symptoms improve before the presence of weight loss or to a greater extent in the context of specific dietary formulations.

Weight loss has positive effects on lung function in subjects with and without asthma. A study of 58 women (24 with asthma, 34 without asthma) enrolled in an intensive 6-month weight loss regimen recorded an average decrease in weight of 20 kg. The FEV_1 and FVC increased significantly (92 mL and 73 mL respectively) for every 10% loss in body weight.[18] Bronchial hyperresponsiveness as measured by response to methacholine was not altered by weight loss, a finding that was reproduced in a study that focused on overweight/obese subjects with asthma.[18,19] However, the conclusions that can be drawn are limited by the sample size and the inclusion of patients without asthma in one of the studies, because this may confound the results.

The role of exercise as an intervention has not been studied extensively. A study that examined the effect of weight loss induced by diet, exercise, or a combination of diet and exercise on asthma symptoms and quality of life noted that exercise alone was insufficient in improving asthma control as measured by the ACQ. Asthma control improved after the dietary and combined interventions with a significant decrease in ACQ scores

Table 1
Changes in markers of asthma control and lung function following dietary weight loss interventions

Study	Design	Population	Intervention	Measured	Changes
Stenius-Aarniala et al,[14] 2000	Randomized controlled trial	Obese asthmatics	14-wk weight reduction program with 8-wk low-calorie diet	Spirometry, PEF Self-reported medication use and exacerbation SGRQ	Improvement in FEV$_1$, FVC, use of rescue medication, and number of exacerbations Sustained improvement in SGRQ
Hakala et al,[15] 2000	Observational	14 obese asthmatics	14 wk weight reduction program with 8-wk low-calorie diet	PEF Spirometry Lung volumes Minute ventilation	Improvement in spirometry, lung volumes, and minute ventilation Decrease in variability of PEF
Aaron et al,[18] 2004	Observation	58 obese women, 24 with asthma	6-mo weight loss program	Spirometry Lung volume Methacholine challenge	Improvement in FEV$_1$, FVC in those who lost weight No change in airway responsiveness
Johnson et al,[16] 2007	Prospective cohort	10 obese moderate persistent asthma	8-wk, alternating-day low-calorie diet	ACQ, mini-AQLQ, ASUI Spirometry PEF	Improvement in all questionnaires and PEF No change in spirometry

Haselkorn et al,[13] 2009	Observational	2396 difficult-to-treat asthmatics	3 groups at 1 y, (lost, maintained, or gained weight)	ATAQ AQLQ Number of steroid bursts	Patients who gained weight had worse questionnaire scores and more steroid bursts Patients who lost weight noted no change
Bafadhel et al,[12] 2010	Observational	151 asthmatics	3 groups at 1 y, (lost, maintained, or gained weight)	Spirometry ACQ	No change in ACQ with weight loss Change in FEV_1 correlates with weight change
Scott et al,[20] 2013	Randomized control trial	46 obese asthmatics	10 wk, diet, exercise, or combination	AQLQ ACQ	AQLQ improved in all groups ACQ only changed in the diet and combination groups
Dias-Junior et al,[19] 2013	Randomized trial	33 moderately obese asthmatics with severe asthma	22 diet and pharmacologic weight loss, 11 control followed at 6 mo	ACQ Rescue medication use Methacholine challenge Spirometry	Improvement in ACQ, FVC, and rescue medication use in weight loss group No change in methacholine challenge response

Abbreviations: ACQ, Asthma Control Questionnaire; AQLQ, Asthma Quality of Life Questionnaire; ASUI, Asthma Symptom Utility Index; ATAQ, Asthma Therapy Assessment Questionnaire; FEV₁, forced expiratory volume in 1 second; FVC, forced vital capacity; PEF, peak expiratory flow; SGRQ, St. George Respiratory Questionaire.

(mean $\pm$ standard deviation, -0.6 ± 0.5, $P = .001$ and -0.5 ± 0.7; $P = .040$). The ability of reductions in weight to improve asthma control as measured by the ACQ score was further shown in a study by Dias-Junior and colleagues.[19] Weight loss and changes in waist circumference and fat mass were significantly greater for the dietary and combined interventions compared with exercise alone and quality of life based on Asthma Quality of Life Questionnaire (AQLQ) scores improved in all groups. The investigators therefore concluded that even a modest amount of weight loss equal to 5% to 10% of total body weight is associated with clinically important improvements in asthma control as defined by a decrease in ACQ score of greater than or equal to 0.5 and in quality of life defined as a change in AQLQ score of greater than or equal to 0.5.[20] These findings are clinically meaningful and suggest that weight loss should be included in the armamentarium of clinical interventions used to manage patients with asthma who are also obese.

SURGICAL INTERVENTION FOR WEIGHT LOSS

Calorie restriction and behavioral modification may be difficult and ineffective in achieving and sustaining a significant amount of weight loss in most morbidly obese patients. Given the increased interest in and prevalence of bariatric surgery as a preferred therapy for morbidly obese adults, we sought to determine whether weight lost via surgical interventions resulted in greater alterations in asthma control and airway hyperresponsiveness (AHR). Early observational studies of bariatric surgery all showed significant improvements in asthma control.[21–26] One of the earliest studies, by Macgregor and Greenberg[21] followed 40 morbidly obese patients with asthma for an average of 4 years (2–11 years) after bariatric surgery. There was an improvement in symptoms or decreased medication use in 90% of patients and 48% of patients reported complete resolution of their asthma.[21] Furthermore, 5 of the 40 patients experienced increased asthma symptoms on regaining weight and all these symptoms resolved with revision of bariatric surgery. A similar study by Dixon and colleagues[22] followed 32 consecutive patients with a physician diagnosis of asthma for a year and administered standard asthma questionnaires after bariatric surgery. During the 1-year follow-up significant decreases in BMI were noted from an average of 45.7 kg/m^2 before surgery to 32.9 kg/m^2 after surgery. The patients were noted concurrently to have an improvement in all asthma-related symptoms assessed by questionnaire, including decreased severity and impact on daily activities, asthma medication use, asthma-related hospitalizations, sleep interruption, and impairments in exercise capacity. Additional observational studies have shown similar improvements in asthma control with complete resolution of asthma symptoms and discontinuation of asthma medicines in 48% to 80% of subjects after bariatric surgery depending on the study.[23–27]

Additional studies have been designed to determine the effect of bariatric surgery on asthma by studying respiratory prescription drug claims.[28] A large cross-sectional study of subjects with asthma in the Swedish Obese Subjects intervention study showed a decrease in asthma-related drug costs in the surgically treated patients, whereas there was an increased cost among patients treated conventionally.[26] A similar study in the United States that followed a cohort of 320 patients for 1 year before and after bariatric surgery also revealed a decrease in the number of prescriptions for asthma-related medications in the first postsurgical year. Only 43% of patients who filled a prescription in the year before surgery filled prescriptions in the year after surgery. Similar results were found when these analyses were restricted to patients with a physician's diagnosis of asthma.[29]

Although these observational studies are intriguing, they largely relied on patient-reported symptoms or medication use as markers of asthma improvement. More recent studies have included objective measures of pulmonary function, AHR, and inflammation. One of the first was a small prospective trial by Maniscalco and colleagues[30] in which 12 obese female subjects with asthma underwent laparoscopic adjustable gastric banding (LAGB) and 10 who did not undergo surgery were followed for 1 year. The intervention group had a significantly improved Asthma Control Test score, FEV_1, and FVC, whereas the control group showed no significant change. The control group had no change in BMI, in contrast with the intervention group whose mean BMI was 45.2 ± 4.7 before surgery, which decreased to 34.8 ± 4.2 after surgery.

Boulet and colleagues[31] completed a study that included 12 patients with asthma undergoing bariatric surgery and 11 not undergoing surgery and noted improvements in ACQ scores and pulmonary function testing. This study also showed that AHR as defined by methacholine challenge (PC20) testing improved after bariatric surgery and that improvement in PC20 was significantly correlated with the change in BMI and C-reactive peptide levels.[32] The change in AHR occurred independently of presence/absence of atopy and metabolic syndrome. Dixon and colleagues[32] followed 23 subjects with asthma for 12 months after bariatric surgery. Bariatric surgery resulted in similar improvements in ACQ scores and FEV_1. There were no significant changes in AHR in the group overall. A post-hoc analysis of surgical subjects divided into 2 groups based on immunoglobulin E (IgE) greater than or less than 100 IU/mL was performed and showed significant improvement in AHR in subjects with IgE levels less than 100 IU/mL but not in those with high IgE levels. These findings suggest that type 2 helper T cell response (TH2) status at baseline may affect response to bariatric surgery. Although patients with TH2 high status had improvements in asthma control and FEV_1 they did not have any changes in AHR. This finding indicates that the TH2 low phenotype may have AHR that is mediated directly by obesity-related mechanisms such as increased cholinergic tone or increased neurogenic inflammation that improves with weight loss and results in decreases in AHR.

We were interested in determining whether the effects on asthma associated with bariatric surgery vary based on surgical technique. A study of 257 patients with asthma who completed a 1-year follow-up survey after bariatric surgery showed an overall reduction in asthma medication use in all patients; however, those who underwent LAGB were only 37% as likely to show improvement in self-reported asthma severity as those with the Roux-en-Y procedure. This finding may be related to the lower percentage of weight loss associated with this procedure. However, change in BMI was not a significant predictor of improvement in asthma medication use on multivariate analysis for all types of bariatric surgery, so the type of surgery may have an impact on asthma-related outcomes.[33] The type of surgery has been shown to have a significant impact on resolution of diabetes even before the presence of a significant amount of weight loss.[34] Perhaps similar mechanisms underlying changes in metabolism are responsible for the disparate findings with regard to improvement in asthma following bariatric surgery. Further evaluation is warranted to determine the best procedure to recommend for a patient undergoing bariatric surgery with significant comorbid asthma.

WEIGHT MANAGEMENT AND IMPROVEMENT IN ASTHMA COMORBIDITIES

Both gastroesophageal reflux disease (GERD) and SDB are often comorbidities with asthma and possibly lead to worsening asthma severity. Treatment of these conditions has been associated with improvements in asthma symptoms in some patients.[35–38] Both GERD and obstructive sleep apnea are also associated with obesity and have been shown to improve with weight loss.[22,23] Macgregor and Greenberg[21] found that although GERD resolved after bariatric surgery in nearly all of the patients who clinically reported symptoms, there was no significant correlation with improvement in asthma, and some patients reported new-onset GERD after surgery and still had improvement in asthma.[22] In a cohort of 257 patients undergoing bariatric surgery, presence of GERD before surgery similarly did not correlate with decreased asthma medication use. On the contrary, the presence of SDB correlated with decreased asthma medication use in univariate analysis but not multivariate analysis.[33] The only study to assess the effects of nonsurgical weight loss interventions on GERD and asthma showed improvements in asthma symptoms despite a lack of change in GERD symptoms.[19] There is a lack of sufficient data to reach conclusions about whether reversal of GERD is the causative factor behind improvements in asthma control with weight loss.

WEIGHT LOSS AND MARKERS OF INFLAMMATION

Adipose tissue plays a key role in mediating systemic inflammation. Obesity results in increased levels of proinflammatory hormones and cytokines, including leptin, resistin, tumor necrosis factor alpha (TNF-α), and interleukin (IL)-6 (**Table 2**).[5,6] The effect of weight loss on systemic inflammation has been shown in several studies, including a reduction in the expression of IL-4, a mediator of TH2 inflammation and other asthma-related gene expression following surgery. Johnson and colleagues[16] noted that weight loss resulted in an improvement in markers of oxidative stress as well as TNF-α and brain-derived neurotrophic factor, which are known mediators of airway inflammation.[6,39] Weight loss in this cohort was additionally associated with improved asthma control and AHR based on decreased variability of PEF. Other studies that evaluated markers of systemic inflammation found no association between weight loss and changes in inflammatory cytokine expression.[12,17,32] It is unclear why weight loss results in variable responses with regard to cytokine expression; however, the study populations were heterogeneous with a variety of weight loss interventions, which may account for the difference. There are 2 studies that reported increases in adiponectin levels with weight loss regardless of whether the weight loss was achieved with surgical or nonsurgical interventions.[20,32]

The correlation between clinical markers of airway inflammation in asthma including fraction of expired nitric oxide (FeNO) and sputum eosinophilia has been examined to determine the effects of obesity on TH2 inflammation. Todd and colleagues[40] reported that BMI was not associated with sputum eosinophilia despite being increased in asthmatics in general. FeNO is not correlated with changes in BMI, suggesting that obesity does not have significant effects on TH2 inflammation.[41] These studies suggest that the effect of obesity may be mediated by non-TH2 inflammatory mechanisms. Weight loss has no effect on FeNO expression[20,31,33] or sputum eosinophilia.[20,32,33] There are 2 studies that show improvements in sputum eosinophilia in a subset of patients.[12,20] The reason for these differential responses has not been delineated but warrants further study. Innate and allergic airway inflammatory responses are likely altered by the presence of obesity and asthma. Dixon and colleagues[32] reported increased cytokine production in stimulated peripheral T-cell cytokine 1 year after bariatric surgery. A study including patients not treated with inhaled corticosteroids yielded similar results, arguing against increased lymphocyte responses being related to decreased antiinflammatory therapy.[41]

Table 2
Changes in inflammatory markers following weight loss via surgical and nonsurgical interventions

Study	Design	Population	Intervention	Measured	Changes
Johnson et al,[16] 2007	Prospective cohort	10 obese moderately persistent asthmatics	8-wk, alternating-day, low-calorie diet	TNF-α BDNP Markers of oxidative stress (8-isoprostane)	All with significant decrease
Maniscalco et al,[30] 2008	Prospective cohort	22 obese asthmatic women	LAGB followed for 1 y	Feno	No significant change
Bafadhel et al,[12] 2010	Observational	151 asthmatics	3 groups at 1 y (lost, maintained, or gained weight)	Feno Sputum eosinophils and neutrophils	No difference in Feno or sputum neutrophils. A decrease in sputum eosinophils in women but not in men who lost weight
Dixon et al,[32] 2011	Prospective	23 obese asthmatic 21 obese nonasthmatic	Bariatric surgery after 1 y	BAL and serum leptin and adiponectin BAL cell count Cytokine production from isolated CD4 cells	Decreased lymphocyte percentage on BAL with increased cytokine response from peripheral T cells No reduction in airway eosinophils No decrease of leptin but increase in BAL and serum adiponectin
Scott et al,[20] 2013	Prospective	46 obese asthmatics	10 wk, diet, exercise, or combination	CRP IL-6 Serum leptin Serum adiponectin Sputum cell count	CRP, IL-6, and adiponectin were unchanged Sputum eosinophils improved in the exercise group only
Dias-Junior et al,[19] 2013	Open randomized trial	33 moderately obese asthmatics with severe asthma	22 diet and pharmacologic weight loss, 11 control at 6 mo	Feno Sputum cell count Serum CRP Serum leptin Serum eotaxin TGFβ-1	There was no difference in any of the measured markers

Abbreviations: BAL, bronchoalveolar lavage; BDNP, brain-derived neurotrophic factor; CRP, C-reactive protein; Feno, fraction of expired nitric oxide; TGFβ-1, transforming growth factor beta-1.

SUMMARY

Although the heterogeneity in definitions of outcome, interventions, and study design make direct comparisons among the reviewed studies challenging, they all support the assertion that weight loss in obese subjects with asthma improves metrics of asthma control and in some cases lung function and AHR. More questions than answers remain and mechanistic studies designed to delineate the pathophysiologic changes that underlie the improvements in asthma control with weight loss are urgently needed.[42–44]

Obesity is likely associated with 2 distinct phenotypes: one driven by traditional forms of TH2 inflammation in which obesity may be a consequence of underlying asthma and associated therapies, and the other that is driven by non-TH2 inflammation that is likely a consequence of the direct effects of obesity-related changes on inflammation.[42,45] In the latter group, AHR may be mediated by mechanisms related directly to obesity, resulting in improvements in hyperresponsiveness with weight loss. It is this group of patients that is most likely to benefit from intensive weight loss strategies or bariatric surgery. Overall, weight loss seems to improve asthma symptoms, decrease medication use, and reduce exacerbations. Therefore weight management strategies should be discussed with overweight or obese patients who have asthma with poor control.

REFERENCES

1. Peters-Golden M, Swern A, Bird SS, et al. Influence of body mass index on the response to asthma controller agents. Eur Respir J 2006;27(3):495–503.
2. Beuther DA, Sutherland ER. Overweight, obesity, and incident asthma: a meta-analysis of prospective epidemiologic studies. Am J Respir Crit Care Med 2007;175(7):661–6.
3. de Oliveira Filho GR, Nicolodi TH, Garcia J, et al. Preanesthetic clinical problems of morbidly obese patients submitted to bariatric surgery: comparison with non-obese patients. Rev Bras Anestesiol 2002;52(2):217–22.
4. Varraso R, Siroux V, Maccario J, et al. Asthma severity is associated with body mass index and early menarche in women. Am J Respir Crit Care Med 2005; 171(4):334–9.
5. Boulet LP. Influence of obesity on the prevalence and clinical features of asthma. Clin Invest Med 2008;31(6):E386–90.
6. Sood A, Shore SA. Adiponectin, leptin, and resistin in asthma: basic mechanisms through population studies. J Allergy (Cairo) 2013;2013:785835.
7. Sood A, Dominic E, Qualls C, et al. Serum adiponectin is associated with adverse outcomes of asthma in men but not in women. Front Pharmacol 2011;2:55.
8. Lugogo NL, Bappanad D, Kraft M. Obesity, metabolic dysregulation and oxidative stress in asthma. Biochim Biophys Acta 2011;1810(11):1120–6.
9. Boulet LP, Tucotte H, Boulet G, et al. Deep inspiration avoidance and airway response to methacholine: Influence of body mass index. Can Respir J 2005; 12(7):371–6.
10. Aaron SD, Vandemheen K, Boulet LP, et al. Overdiagnosis of asthma in obese and nonobese adults. CMAJ 2008;179(11):1121–31.
11. Lugogo NL, Hollingsworth J, Howell DL, et al. Alveolar macrophages from overweight/obese subjects with asthma demonstrate a proinflammatory phenotype. Am J Respir Crit Care Med 2012;186(5):404–11.
12. Bafadhel M, Singapuri A, Terry S, et al. Body mass and fat mass in refractory asthma: an observational 1 year follow-up study. J Allergy (Cairo) 2010;2010:251758.

13. Haselkorn T, Fish J, Chipps B, et al. Effect of weight change on asthma-related health outcomes in patients with severe or difficult-to-treat asthma. Respir Med 2009;103(2):274–83.

14. Stenius-Aarniala B, Poussa T, Kvarnstrom J, et al. Immediate and long term effects of weight reduction in obese people with asthma: randomised controlled study. BMJ 2000;320(7238):827–32.

15. Hakala K, Stenius-Aarniala B, Sovijarvi A. Effects of weight loss on peak flow variability, airways obstruction, and lung volumes in obese patients with asthma. Chest 2000;118(5):1315–21.

16. Johnson JB, Summer W, Cutler RG, et al. Alternate day calorie restriction improves clinical findings and reduces markers of oxidative stress and inflammation in overweight adults with moderate asthma. Free Radic Biol Med 2007;42(5): 665–74.

17. Hernandez Romero A, Matta Campos J, Mora Nieto A, et al. Clinical symptom relief in obese patients with persistent moderate asthma secondary to decreased obesity. Rev Alerg Mex 2008;55(3):103–11.

18. Aaron SD, Fergusson D, Dent R, et al. Effect of weight reduction on respiratory function and airway reactivity in obese women. Chest 2004;125(6):2046–52.

19. Dias-Junior SA, Reis M, de Carvalho-Pinto RM, et al. Effects of weight loss on asthma control in obese patients with severe asthma. Eur Respir J 2013;43(5):1368–77.

20. Scott HA, Gibson PG, Garg ML, et al. Dietary restriction and exercise improve airway inflammation and clinical outcomes in overweight and obese asthma: a randomized trial. Clin Exp Allergy 2013;43(1):36–49.

21. Macgregor AM, Greenberg RA. Effect of surgically induced weight loss on asthma in the morbidly obese. Obes Surg 1993;3(1):15–21.

22. Dixon JB, Chapman L, O'Brien P. Marked improvement in asthma after Lap-Band surgery for morbid obesity. Obes Surg 1999;9(4):385–9.

23. Spivak H, Hewitt MF, Onn A, et al. Weight loss and improvement of obesity-related illness in 500 U.S. patients following laparoscopic adjustable gastric banding procedure. Am J Surg 2005;189(1):27–32.

24. Dhabuwala A, Cannan RJ, Stubbs RS. Improvement in co-morbidities following weight loss from gastric bypass surgery. Obes Surg 2000;10(5):428–35.

25. O'Brien PE, Dixon JB, Brown W, et al. The laparoscopic adjustable gastric band (Lap-Band): a prospective study of medium-term effects on weight, health and quality of life. Obes Surg 2002;12(5):652–60.

26. Brancatisano A, Wahlroos S, Brancatisano R. Improvement in comorbid illness after placement of the Swedish adjustable gastric band. Surg Obes Relat Dis 2008; 4(3 Suppl):S39–46.

27. Hewitt S, Humerfelt S, Sovik TT, et al. Long-term improvements in pulmonary function 5 years after bariatric surgery. Obes Surg 2014;24(5):705–11.

28. Narbro K, Agren G, Jonsson E, et al. Pharmaceutical costs in obese individuals: comparison with a randomly selected population sample and long-term changes after conventional and surgical treatment: the SOS intervention study. Arch Intern Med 2002;162(18):2061–9.

29. Sikka N, Wegienka G, Havstad S, et al. Respiratory medication prescriptions before and after bariatric surgery. Ann Allergy Asthma Immunol 2010;104(4):326–30.

30. Maniscalco M, Zedda A, Faraone S, et al. Weight loss and asthma control in severely obese asthmatic females. Respir Med 2008;102(1):102–8.

31. Boulet LP, Turcotte H, Martin J, et al. Effect of bariatric surgery on airway response and lung function in obese subjects with asthma. Respir Med 2012; 106(5):651–60.

32. Dixon AE, Reis M, de Carvalho-Pinto RM, et al. Effects of obesity and bariatric surgery on airway hyperresponsiveness, asthma control, and inflammation. J Allergy Clin Immunol 2011;128(3):508–15.e1–2.

33. Reddy RC, Baptist AP, Fan Z, et al. The effects of bariatric surgery on asthma severity. Obes Surg 2011;21(2):200–6.

34. Araia M, Wood M, Krool J, et al. Resolution of diabetes after bariatric surgery among predominantly African-American patients: race has no effect in remission of diabetes after bariatric surgery. Obes Surg 2014;24(6):835–40.

35. Puthalapattu S, Ioachimescu OC. Asthma and obstructive sleep apnea: clinical and pathogenic interactions. J Investig Med 2014;62(4):665–75.

36. Prasad B, Nyenhuis SM, Weaver TE. Obstructive sleep apnea and asthma: associations and treatment implications. Sleep Med Rev 2014;18(2):165–71.

37. Kiljander TO, Laitinen JO. The prevalence of gastroesophageal reflux disease in adult asthmatics. Chest 2004;126(5):1490–4.

38. Chan WW, Chiou E, Obstein KL, et al. The efficacy of proton pump inhibitors for the treatment of asthma in adults: a meta-analysis. Arch Intern Med 2011;171(7):620–9.

39. Lommatzsch M, Schloetcke K, Klotz J, et al. Brain-derived neurotrophic factor in platelets and airflow limitation in asthma. Am J Respir Crit Care Med 2005;171(2):115–20.

40. Todd DC, Armstrong S, D'Silva L, et al. Effect of obesity on airway inflammation: a cross-sectional analysis of body mass index and sputum cell counts. Clin Exp Allergy 2007;37(7):1049–54.

41. McLachlan CR, Poulton R, Car G, et al. Adiposity, asthma, and airway inflammation. J Allergy Clin Immunol 2007;119(3):634–9.

42. Sideleva O, Black K, Dixon AE. Effects of obesity and weight loss on airway physiology and inflammation in asthma. Pulm Pharmacol Ther 2013;26(4):455–8.

43. Adeniyi FB, Young T. Weight loss interventions for chronic asthma. Cochrane Database Syst Rev 2012;(7):CD009339.

44. Moreira A, Bonini M, Garcia-Larsen V, et al. Weight loss interventions in asthma: EAACI evidence-based clinical practice guideline (part I). Allergy 2013;68(4):425–39.

45. Lugogo NL, Kraft M, Dixon AE. Does obesity produce a distinct asthma phenotype? J Appl Physiol (1985) 2010;108(3):729–34.

Novel Therapeutic Strategies for Adult Obese Asthmatics

Angela L. Linderholm, PhD[a], Jennifer M. Bratt, PhD[a],
Gertrud U. Schuster, PhD[b,c], Amir A. Zeki, MD, MAS[a],
Nicholas J. Kenyon, MD, MAS[a,*]

KEYWORDS

- Severe asthma • L-Arginine • Nitric oxide • Metformin • Statins • Obesity

KEY POINTS

- In the future, treatment regimens for obese, adult asthmatics may include several interventions that interfere with pathways common to several metabolic and nutritional disorders.
- The diabetic drug, metformin, could decrease inflammatory mediators of asthma by improving insulin sensitivity and altering adenosine monophosphate–activated protein kinase (AMPK).
- The cholesterol-lowering class of medications, statins, could have beneficial effects on both airway inflammation and structural remodeling in asthma.
- L-Arginine supplementation may benefit a subset of severe asthmatic patients with impaired nitric oxide (NO) synthase function in the lung.

INTRODUCTION

Adult obese patients with worsening asthma despite appropriate controller drug therapy are extraordinarily complicated to manage and treat. For example, consider a 40-year-old woman with a medical history notable for adult-onset nonallergic

Disclosure: The authors appreciate ongoing support from the National Institutes of Health (T32 HL07013 [J.M. Bratt], K08 HL076415 [A. Zeki], and HL105573, AI097354 [N.J. Kenyon]). The authors have no other disclosures.
[a] Division of Pulmonary, Critical Care and Sleep Medicine, Department of Internal Medicine, University of California, Davis, 4150 V Street, Suite 3100, Davis, CA, USA; [b] Nutrition Department, University of California, Davis, 430 West Health Sciences Drive, Davis, CA, USA; [c] Immunity and Diseases Prevention Unit, Western Human Nutrition Research Center, United States Department of Agriculture (USDA), Agricultural Research Services (ARS), 430 West Health Sciences Drive, Davis, CA, USA
* Corresponding author. Division of Pulmonary, Critical Care and Sleep Medicine, University of California, Davis, 451 Health Sciences Drive, GBSF, Suite 6510, Davis, CA 95616.
E-mail address: njkenyon@ucdavis.edu

asthma, obesity, diabetes mellitus, and sleep apnea whose course has been punctuated by several emergency department admissions in the past year. She already requires continuous oral prednisone and 4-drug therapy for her asthma. How should such a patient be evaluated and treated for the foreseeable future? Although asthma is a complex syndrome that affects an estimated 26 million people in the United States, there are gaps in the recognition and management of asthmatic subgroups. Extrapolating results from short-term, randomized clinical trials to a broad, heterogeneous population of asthmatics treated in community settings is fraught with difficulty and can result in repeated trial-and-error therapeutic interventions. The ability to recognize different asthma phenotypes, to adapt and integrate care when comorbidities exist, and adopt new treatments is still lacking. Although published guidelines, including the National Asthma Education and Prevention Program Expert Panel Report 3 and the World Health Organization Global Initiative for Asthma, present stepwise evaluation and therapeutic recommendations for chronic persistent asthma management, they do not outline coherent plans for the care of adult-onset obese asthmatics.

This article proposes alternative approaches that may prove to be future treatments for adult obese asthmatics who do not respond to the standard controller asthma therapies of inhaled corticosteroids, bronchodilators, and antileukotriene (LT) drugs. Parallels are drawn between seemingly disparate therapeutics through their common signaling pathways (**Fig. 1**). Specifically, how metformin and statins potentially improve airway inflammation through activation of AMPK, a key regulator of cellular metabolism and energy production, and through their effects on NO is described. In addition, nutritional supplements, such as L-arginine, omega-3 (n-3) fatty acids, and other minerals and vitamins that are currently studied and may potentially be used in combination with conventional therapies are described.

METFORMIN, INSULIN RESISTANCE, AND ASTHMA

The metabolic syndrome with insulin resistance may characterize subsets of asthmatics more than is recognized. The relationship between obesity, insulin resistance, and asthma has been clearly established; however, the mechanisms by which they influence the pathogenesis of asthma is unclear.[1] Metformin is a biguanide class oral antidiabetic drug used to treat type 2 diabetes mellitus and insulin resistance. Although metformin reduces glucose production in the liver through inhibition of gluconeogenesis, the precise mechanisms are unknown and it may have differing modalities in different cell types. Metformin may indirectly activate AMPK by increasing AMP:ATP ratios through mild but specific inhibition of the mitochondrial respiratory chain complex I in hepatocytes, skeletal muscle, endothelial cells, pancreatic B cells, and neurons.[2] Peroxynitrite, generated by inhibition of complex I, activates AMPK through a c-Src and PI3K–dependent pathway in bovine aortic endothelial cells.[3] Metformin also directly activates AMPK through the inhibition of AMP deaminase in isolated skeletal muscle.[4] In the lung, metformin up-regulates AMPK expression and activity and diminishes proinflammatory cytokine secretion in human bronchial epithelial cells, down-regulating IκB kinase activity and inhibiting nuclear factor (NF)-κB.[5]

Obese asthmatics are less responsive to typical asthma controller therapy possibly because of contributing factors, such as an increased proinflammatory environment, that blunt the efficacy of treatment,[6] yet there have been studies that have shown no difference in induced sputum eosinophils, a biomarker of airway inflammation, between obese and lean asthmatics.[7,8] In a study of obese and lean asthmatics by Desai and colleagues,[9] however, there were similarities in sputum eosinophil counts between the 2 groups but an increase in interleukin-5 (IL-5), a mediator of eosinophil

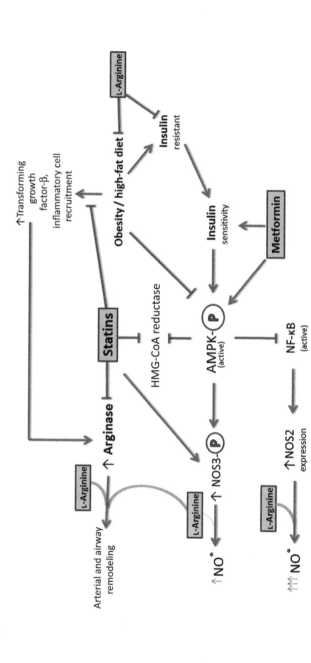

Fig. 1. Potential therapeutics for obese, adult asthmatics described in this review modulate pathways common to several metabolic and nutritional disorders, allowing for the treatment of several comorbidities by targeting their common dysfunction as opposed to individual symptoms. Direct targets include AMPK, which regulates numerous cellular metabolic pathways involved in energy storage, and NOS3, which modulates vascular and bronchial smooth muscle tone. HMG-CoA, hydroxymethylglutaryl–coenzyme A.

activation, in the sputum and increased eosinophil accumulation in the submucosal layer of the obese asthmatic group.

The results from a study using a high-fat diet–induced obese mouse model (male C57BL6/J) of allergic airway inflammation are in agreement with patient observations. Although eosinophil numbers in the bronchoalveolar lavage (BAL) from allergen-challenged obese mice were decreased compared with their lean counterparts, the levels of infiltrated eosinophils in the lung tissue were higher in the obese mice. Treatment of these allergen-challenged obese mice with metformin reduced tissue eosinophil infiltration and increased the number of cells in the BAL fluid suggest differing modes of regulation for eosinophil migration and function between obese and lean asthmatics, possibly through decreased NF-κB activation.[10] Another mouse study using lean BALB/C female mice demonstrated that metformin decreases eosinophilic inflammation, peribronchial fibrosis, and mucin secretion coupled with increased ratios of activated phospho-AMPK to total AMPK and decreased oxidative stress as measured by the ratio of reduced to oxidized glutathione.[11]

Metformin can also increase NO synthase 3 (NOS3) dependent production of NO and improve endothelial function through AMPK-dependent positive regulation of NOS3 activity and inhibition of NOS3 negative regulators. Treatment of endothelial cell lines and mice with metformin increases AMPK-dependent NOS3 phosphorylation at the regulatory site Ser1177/1179 and NO production.[12–14] NOS3 activity is negatively regulated through phosphorylation of Thr495 by protein kinase C-β (PKCβ), which is up-regulated in human asthmatics and patients with insulin resistance.[15] Pharmacologic inhibition of PKCβ in endothelial cells freshly isolated from diabetics decreases basal levels of Thr495 phosphorylated NOS3 and improved insulin-mediated signaling of NOS3. Overall NOS expression and activity are also reduced in murine models of allergic inflammation and human asthmatics.[16–18] Overexpression of NOS3 in a mouse model of allergic asthma attenuates airway inflammation and airway hyperresponsiveness, possibly acting through increased levels of S-nitrosothiols in the lung or decreased interferon-γ, IL-5, or IL-10.[19] Further studies are necessary to uncover whether NOS3 could be regulated by metformin in models of asthma or asthmatics.

These findings suggest that introducing metformin in conjunction with standard asthma controller therapy could prove beneficial for outcomes in obese asthmatics by modulation of NOS3 activity or other AMPK-dependent metabolic signaling pathways.

ASTHMA, THE MEVALONATE PATHWAY, AND THE STATIN DRUGS

The statin class of drugs inhibits the enzyme, hydroxymethylglutaryl–coenzyme A reductase (HMGCR), which is the rate-limiting step in cholesterol and isoprenoid biosynthesis in the mevalonate (MVA) pathway.[20] Isoprenoids include pyrophosphate lipid molecules (eg, farnesylpyrophosphate [FPP] and geranylgeranylpyrophosphate [GGPP]) that are necessary for post-translational modification of numerous intracellular proteins, including small G-proteins, or GTPases (eg, Rho, Ras, and Rac). GTPases require prenyl tethering to the membrane to maintain proximity to the appropriate transmembrane receptors and signaling transduction machinery. Limiting the availability of the isoprenoid substrate reduces the total amount of GTPase available for activation, potentially dampening cytokine and chemokine signal transduction and the responses that lead to cellular hypertrophy and inflammation.[21]

Statins' effect on isoprenylated GTPases is a mechanism that may be of particular interest in targeting the obese asthmatic population because translational studies in obese (ob/ob, leptin –/–) mice exposed to allergen have indicated increased activity of the GTPase, RhoA, in airway epithelial cells and airway smooth muscle. Increased RhoA activity has been implicated in airway smooth muscle hyperreactivity and hypertrophy. GGPP synthase (GGPPS) expression, the enzyme upstream of FPP and GGPP synthesis, is also increased in obese (ob/ob) mice. Because RhoA requires prenylation by GGPP for activation, the use of statins to manipulate the MVA pathway may have further implications for airway hyperreactivity and remodeling, 2 key features in asthma.[22,23]

Statins may also regulate L-arginine metabolism and NO production. In addition to being induced by Th2 cytokines IL-4 and IL-13, arginase 1 or 2 expression can be induced via a RhoA/Rho associated protein kinase (ROCK)–mediated pathway. Endothelial cell RhoA/ROCK can be indirectly activated by reactive oxygen and nitrogen species, such as H_2O_2 and $ONOO^-$, via protein kinase C. Insulin resistance and diabetes increases the production of these oxidative species through several sources, including uncoupled mitochondrial complex 1, mitochondrial NOS (mtNOS), and NOS3.

RhoA-dependent activation of ROCK increases arginase 1 expression in aortas and livers of streptozotocin-induced diabetic rats. Arginase activity depletes intracellular and plasma L-arginine, further reducing endothelium-derived NO production and promoting additional NOS uncoupling. This effect on endothelial NO production is reversible, however, with administration of statins, ROCK inhibitor Y-27632, or L-citrulline.[24–26] The inhibitory effect of simvastatin on arginase expression and activity has also been observed in the airways of mice, in a model of allergic inflammation, although its mechanism of action has not been determined, because statins also inhibit the expression of IL-13 in airway epithelial cells.[27,28] Statin-dependent reduction in circulating ADMA further aids production of NO by the NOS enzymes and reduces NOS uncoupling. Thus, simvastatin (and potentially other statins) can function to improve dysfunctional NO metabolism in asthmatic, inflamed lungs.

Statins and AMPK collectively engage in crosstalk that regulates NOS3 activity. Treatment of human endothelial cells with statins results in time- and dose-dependent increases in phosphorylated AMPK, followed by AMPK-dependent phosphorylation of NOS3 at Ser1177.[29] These results were confirmed in the aorta and myocardium of mice orally administered atorvastatin.[30] Independent of statin administration, AMPK activation also inhibited HMGCR by phosphorylation of the Ser871/Ser872 site in cultured rat hepatocytes and human endothelial cells.[31,32]

Statins applied to murine models of allergen-induced airway inflammation reduce inflammatory cell influx, Th2 cytokine production, ADMA levels, airway hyperreactivity, and airway remodeling.[33–36] Specific inhibition of geranylgeranyltransferase by GGTI-2133 reduces airway hyperreactivity, whereas farnesyltransferase inhibition increases inflammation and airway hyperreactivity. This indicates that the effect of statins on airway smooth muscle is dependent on reduced isoprenylation of RhoA by GGPP and the therapeutic effect of statins, at least in allergic airway disease, is through its effects on geranylgeranylation (ie, RhoA), not farnesylation.[37]

In the authors' severe asthma clinics, female-predominant severe asthmatics with a mean body mass index (BMI) of greater than or equal to 30 were found to benefit from statin treatment. Median statin use for 1 year added to standard inhaler treatment was associated with a higher asthma control test score, indicating improved asthma symptoms.[38] Because this is the only study the authors are aware of that evaluates statin use in obese severe asthmatics, clinical application is precluded absent randomized clinical trials to test this observation.

Although data are limited in obese asthmatics, studies by Chiba and Zeki et al.,[33,34] support the biological plausibility for the role of MVA metabolism and statins in mitigating asthma in this subgroup. Nonatopic adult-onset asthmatics, especially individuals with the confounding characteristics of obesity and metabolic syndrome, tend to be more severe and refractory to current therapies. These additional comorbidities contribute to systemic inflammation, insulin resistance, and reduced lung function originating from inflammation and mechanical stress derived from increased visceral mass. Statins may address many of these comorbidities; statins reduce proinflammatory signaling by RhoA/ROCK, increase NO production and reduce the production of oxidative species by uncoupled NOS enzyme, and activate AMPK, reversing insulin resistance. Therefore, the authors believe that future experiments in animal models and clinical trials with adult-onset asthmatics with obesity should evaluate the potential therapeutic role of statins and/or statin with L-arginine combination treatment.

L-ARGININE AND ASTHMA

L-Arginine is a substrate in protein synthesis, a molecular component for the conversion of ammonia to urea in the urea cycle, and the substrate in several diverse enzymatic pathways, including the synthesis of NO, creatine, agmatine, ornithine, glutamate, proline, polyamine, and dimethylarginines, including asymmetric dimethylarginine (ADMA).

Dietary supplementation of amino acid formulations is common practice among healthy individuals and those with chronic illnesses. The semi-essential amino acid, L-arginine, has been reported to confer beneficial effects in various small studies of surgery, trauma, and infectious and noninfectious inflammation. Direct infusion of L-arginine to the peripheral or pulmonary arterial beds has been tested in acute and chronic disease states, including coronary heart disease, preeclampsia, and myocardial infarction, because of its bronchodilator and vasodilator actions.[39–41] L-Arginine can also be used as a primary therapeutic in sickle cell disease patients with acute chest syndrome, where deficiency in NOS3-derived NO contributes to red cell sickling and vasoconstriction,[42] augmenting NO production and improving outcomes in this disease.

Factors that regulate the output of NO in the airway, endothelium, and adipose tissues of asthmatics include the concentration of L-arginine, the metabolic precursor of NO, and ADMA, an endogenous NOS inhibitor. NO is primarily derived from the oxidative deamination of L-arginine and O_2 into NO and L-citrulline by the NOS family of enzymes. This family includes NOS1 (neuronal NOS), NOS2 (inducible NOS), and NOS3 (endothelial NOS). NOS is also present in mitochondria and referred to as mtNOS but is a variant of NOS1.[43] Depletion of L-arginine can cause the NOS isoforms to produce superoxide ($\bullet O_2^-$) in a process referred to as *uncoupling* that results in the transfer of an electron from NADPH to oxygen instead of L-arginine.[44,45] NO and superoxide ($\bullet O_2^-$) can combine to form peroxynitrite ($ONOO^-$). Thus, reduced L-arginine availability to NOS enzymes can have the double effect of reducing NO output and producing oxidative and nitrosative species.

Initial studies using DNA microarray analysis in mouse models of allergen-induced inflammation identified the arginase enzymes as potential "asthma signature genes." Arginase 1 and arginase 2 catalyze the hydrolysis of L-arginine to ornithine and urea. Increased arginase activity in asthmatics and particularly obese asthmatics is important both for the downstream products of arginase activity, including proline and polyamines, which contribute to airway remodeling and cellular proliferation, and its capacity to regulate the availability of L-arginine to the NOS enzymes by substrate depletion. Analysis of lung tissue of asthmatic subjects confirmed that increased arginase 1 expression correlated with additional effects of increased serum arginase activity and decreased plasma L-arginine compared with controls.[17,46] Further analysis based on patient subpopulation revealed that serum arginase 1 level in nonatopic asthmatics was further amplified compared with atopic asthmatics.

Animal models of allergic airway inflammation have shown that inhibition of arginase ameliorated lung inflammation; reduced airway and peribronchial eosinophilia; and decreased production of Th2 proinflammatory cytokines, IL-4 and IL-13, and eotaxins. Arginase inhibition reduced characteristics of airway remodeling, including goblet cell hyperplasia, airway smooth muscle proliferation, and subepithelial collagen accumulation. Airway hyperreactivity and airway maximal contraction were also reduced.[47–50] In lieu of arginase inhibition, supplementation with oral or aerosolized L-arginine produced comparable results, indicating that the driving force for these improvements was maintaining adequate levels of L-arginine.[51]

Increased arginase activity in the obese, nonatopic asthmatic subpopulation may be derived from sources beyond the lung. Obese subjects have heightened expression of arginase 1 (4.5-fold) in circulating mononuclear cells compared with normal-weight subjects.[52] Exposure to high levels of insulin causes endothelial cells to have increased arginase 2 activity that leads to the uncoupling of NOS3 and increased inflammatory cell adhesion via soluble intercellular cellular adhesion molecule 1. Abrogation of these effects can be achieved through arginase inhibition.[53] Hyperglycemic rats have increased arginase 1 and arginase 2 expression in muscle arteriole beds, which inhibit the vasodilation resulting from increased flow. Inhibition of arginase reverses the arteriole flow impedance.[54] In these models, the beneficial effects of arginase inhibition include mitigation of hypertension, insulin resistance, and systemic inflammation.

In an ongoing phase II study (NCT01841281), the authors are examining a subset of adult severe asthmatics who are predominantly overweight/obese and female. The go-to biomarkers that are indicative of asthma do not necessarily apply for this obese, late-onset population, because this subset is nonatopic (low circulating IgE) and exhibit low exhaled NO, which inversely correlates with BMI and deceptively low sputum eosinophilia.[55] Shifts in NO metabolism are indicative of the vascular dysfunction relating to obesity, and the changes in exhaled NO may represent corresponding changes in the lung.[9] The authors hypothesize that this subset of asthmatics will respond favorably to L-arginine supplementation in addition to their standard therapy because in obese asthmatics, the age of asthma onset seems to dictate how they respond to controller therapies, whether their obesity is causative or a comorbid condition.

ADMA AND PHOSPHODIESTERASE INHIBITION

NO production by the NOS enzymes can be inhibited by endogenous competitive inhibitor, ADMA, which can uncouple NOS enzymes, producing superoxide. ADMA is derived from the posttranslational modification of L-arginine by protein-arginine methyltransferase type 1.[56] The lung is a major source of protein-bound asymmetric dimethylarginine with greater than 3-fold higher levels of bound ADMA compared with heart, kidney, or liver tissue, and an estimated 1.4% of arginine residues present in lung proteins asymmetrically dimethylated.[57] Proteolytic degradation of these proteins releases methylarginases to the free amino acid pool[58,59] where they can be enzymatically converted into L-citrulline and dimethylamine by the dimethylarginine dimethylaminohydrolase (DDAH) enzymes or excreted in the urine.[60]

The lung arginine:ADMA ratio is significantly altered in asthmatics compared with nonasthmatics, with sputum ADMA inversely correlating to exhaled NO.[61] Increased plasma ADMA has been observed in numerous disease states, including pulmonary arteriole hypertension, chronic obstructive pulmonary disease (COPD), cardiovascular disease, and diabetes mellitus.[61–63] The subgroup consisting of obese, nonatopic asthmatics, independent of other confounding metabolic risk factors, may have significantly increased levels of plasma ADMA and reduced L-arginine:ADMA ratio due to obesity alone.[64] Other potentiating factors, such as insulin resistance, even in normotensive individuals, also correlate with increased ADMA.[65,66]

Mouse models of allergic airway inflammation have given further insight into the role of ADMA metabolism in disease. Allergen exposed mice, like human asthmatics, have significantly increased levels of ADMA in their serum and BALF[67] and further examination revealed increased synthesis of ADMA in alveolar epithelial cells and macrophages and reduced expression of ADMA catabolic enzyme, DDAH2, in airway epithelial cells compared with control mice.[67] Altering ADMA degradation by overexpressing DDAH1 reduced markers of inflammation, including eosinophilia, Th2 cytokines IL-4 and IL-13, arginase, and IgE.[68]

DDAH2 expression is regulated by intracellular cyclic adenosine monophosphate (cAMP) concentration via protein kinase A (PKA)-dependent phosphorylation of the transcription factor, cAMP response element-binding (CREB) protein. PKA activation is mediated by cAMP binding to PKA-regulatory subunits, resulting in the release of active PKA, which can phosphorylate numerous targets, including CREB, which require phosphorylation to facilitate binding to the CRE domains upstream of the human DDAH2 gene. Inhibiting cAMP to AMP conversion through the use of phosphodiesterase (PDE) 3/4 inhibitors increases catabolism of the endogenous NOS inhibitor, ADMA, and increasing NOS3 activity in endothelium and alveolar macrophages.[69,70] Activation of PKA by PDE4 inhibitors may also target RhoA pathways. PKA-dependent RhoA phosphorylation inhibits RhoA activation, and phosphorylation of guanine nucleotide dissociation inhibitor (GDI) by PKA enhances GDI binding to RhoA, deactivating it.[71] Because the RhoA/ROCK pathway also regulates expression of arginase, this pathway may further alleviate the depletion of L-arginine and NOS uncoupling.[26,72]

PDE4 inhibitors tested in murine models of chronic allergic airway inflammation reduce airway eosinophilia, inflammatory cell recruitment, matrix metalloprotease 9 activity, fibroblast migration and hypercontractility, and subepithelial collagen deposition.[73,74] For patient use, second-generation PDE4 inhibitors for treatment of COPD have completed multiple randomized clinical trials, noting improvement in prebronchodilator forced expiratory volume in the first second of expiration, with limited side effects, including nausea, diarrhea, headaches, and weight loss. In combination with other asthma control therapies, the use of PDE4 inhibitors to treat severe, obese asthmatics, especially those with measurably heightened plasma ADMA levels, may provide therapeutic benefits.

The potential treatment options reviewed in this section are united by the common principle that decreasing NOS uncoupling has significant clinical benefit in the subgroup of obese, nonatopic asthmatics in which the compounding factors of obesity, endothelial dysfunction, metabolic syndrome, and lung inflammation all contribute to perpetuating NOS dysfunction. These treatments approach the issue of deficient NO production from numerous directions. Supplementation with L-arginine bolsters the L-arginine:ADMA ratio, effectively outcompeting the NOS inhibitor molecule based on enzyme saturation and directly addressing the issue of limited substrate uncoupling NOS enzymes. Arginase inhibition indirectly produces the same effect, increasing both intracellular and plasma L-arginine availability and increasing the L-arginine: ADMA ratio. Finally, inhibition of PDE4 increases ADMA catabolism by decreasing cAMP turnover and subsequently increasing expression of DDAH2. The uncoupling of NOS by ADMA and/or substrate depletion results in the production of oxidative and nitrosative species in the airways, inflammatory cells, endothelial cells and adipose tissue, contributing to the progression of disease.

VITAMINS AND OMEGA-3 POLYUNSATURATED FATTY ACIDS: OTHER POTENTIAL CONSIDERATION IN ASTHMA AND OBESITY

The bioavailability of fat-soluble vitamins A, D, and E in asthmatic patients has not been intensely explored but it can have an impact on obese asthmatic patients because body fat likely acts as a reservoir for storage of fat-soluble vitamins. Although more research must be done to evaluate the adequate status of these vitamins in obese asthmatic patients, a summary of these vitamins and omega-3 polyunsaturated fatty acid (PUFAs) and their impact on asthma is included.

Recent epidemiologic studies point to an inverse relationship between vitamin A levels and severity of asthma.[75,76] Vitamin A affects a broad array of immune responses through retinoic acid (RA), its major oxidative metabolite. Previous data indicate that vitamin A deficiency can impair immune function, whereas excess RA induces inflammatory disorders. Vitamin A or RA limits the differentiation of naïve T cells to T-helper cell (Th)1 by reducing IL-12, INF-γ, and NF-κB signaling, resulting in the increase of Th2-mediated processes. RA can oppose Th17 cell commitment by increasing TGF-β signaling and reducing the expression of IL-6 receptor, whereas excess vitamin A results in the induction of different subsets of Foxp3$^+$ regulatory T (Treg) cells and their mediated processes.[77] RA has also been shown to inhibit eosinophilic and basophilic differentiation and regulate IgA and IgG production in response to T-cell–dependent antigens. Results from studies in mice and rodents suggest strongly that adequate vitamin A status is the key for maintaining a balance of well-regulated T-cell differentiation and function.

The clinicaltrials.gov web site cites more than 25 asthma studies that are ongoing with vitamin D. Vitamin D supplementation and asthma have been studied for years and the conflicting findings are likely due to differences in study design, sample size, and method for assessing vitamin D status through measuring levels of 25-hydroxyvitamin D (25(OH)D).[78,79] Potential beneficial effects of 1,25-dihydroxyvitamin D (calcitriol) synthesized by bronchial epithelial cells include increasing antimicrobial peptide production by facilitating Toll-like receptor signaling, regulation of the inflammatory response, airway remodeling, and respiratory muscle function. Circulating 25(OH)D can suppress IL-17– and IL-4–mediated expression of IL-13 and shift the Th1/Th2 balance toward Th2 dominance. These controversial functions may be due to the direct effect of vitamin D on CD4$^+$ T cells by promoting an IL-10 secreting population of Treg cells.[79] In addition, supplementation of calcitriol has been associated with decreases in body fat mass and improved insulin sensitivity in obese people.[80] Despite supplementation of vitamin D, large populations remain vitamin D deficient. This could apply to the adult obese asthmatic population, because the bioavailability seems to be decreased with increased body fat mass.

Although vitamin A and D exert most of their affects through the binding of nuclear receptors and regulating of gene transcription, vitamin C and E act as potent antioxidants. Deficiencies in vitamin C and other plasma antioxidants are associated with lung disease and case-control and cross-sectional studies suggest that vitamin C supplementation may decrease asthma severity and exacerbation frequency through antioxidant mechanisms.[81] Vitamin E supplementation in asthmatics has been shown to help stabilize lung epithelia membranes and protect against ozone-induced membrane injury by interrupting lipid peroxidation.[82] Increased levels of vitamin E are associated with less allergic skin sensitization, lower IgE secretion, and suppressed neutrophil recruitment. Vitamin E supplementation in animal studies improves vasodilation and decreases oxidation of LDL through increased antioxidants levels in the vasculature. Randomized controlled clinical trials of supplemental vitamin E in asthmatics have not, however, consistently demonstrated that higher intake of vitamin E reduces asthma events.[83]

Several clinical studies have been designed to test the hypothesis that diets supplemented with the omega-3 PUFAs, eicosapentanoic acid (EPA) and docosahexaenoic acid (DHA), the major component of fish oil, ameliorate the development of asthma or improve asthma outcomes.[84] In the context of asthma, in the obese patient subgroup, intervention trials with n-3 PUFAs show beneficial effects in patients with type 2 diabetes mellitus and cardiovascular disease.[85,86] EPA has an impact on inflammatory signaling by competitively inhibiting enzymatic pathways that convert arachidonic acid (AA) to potent proinflammatory 4-series LTs and 2-series prostaglandins (PGs), mediated by 5-lipoxygenase and cyclooxygenase (COX). EPA may also inhibit IgE production through COX.[87] In addition, EPA is metabolized to less inflammatory 5-series LTs and 3-series PGs and potent anti-inflammatory mediators, resolvins of the E-series (RvE1 and Rv3). The effects of DHA are distinct from EPA; DHA can decrease transcription of AA metabolizing enzymes, such as COX-2, by inhibiting NF-κB activation. DHA can also be converted into anti-inflammatory mediators, including the resolvins of the D-series (RvD1, RvD2, RvD3, and RvD4), docosatrienes, and protectins.[88] Results of the studies testing effects of n-3 PUFAs on asthma pathogenesis over the past 20 years have been conflicting and at least 1 meta-analysis determined that n-3 PUFAs does not affect asthma outcomes.[84] There is a consensus, however, that the total number of subjects in these trials is insufficient to make firm conclusions about the effects of the supplements.

FUTURE CONSIDERATIONS/SUMMARY

Controller drug therapies for asthma may be partly or wholly ineffective in adult obese, nonatopic asthma patients, leaving them poorly controlled and exposed to adverse drug side effects, such as relative adrenal insufficiency, osteoporosis, and more frequent respiratory viral infections. One approach to therapy does not fit all and physicians must demonstrate a willingness to try several treatment alternatives. The authors recommend that asthmatic patients not appropriately responding to controller drug therapy be re-evaluated. Adult obese, nonallergic asthmatics may have concomitant conditions that potentiate systemic inflammation; in turn, they may respond to treatment targeted at these associated conditions. Patients with the metabolic syndrome, hypercholesterolemia, and diabetes treated with either metformin or the statin drugs may find benefit for their asthma as well as their metabolic derangements. Although firm recommendations cannot be made until further studies are performed, these medications, L-arginine, omega-3 fatty acids, and other nutritional supplements are exciting considerations for future treatment of asthma. A move toward more targeted therapies for asthma subgroups is needed, and, biologically, these therapies account for and treat the comorbidities associated with obese, nonatopic asthmatic patients.

REFERENCES

1. Weiss ST. Obesity: insight into the origins of asthma. Nat Immunol 2005;6(6): 537–9.

2. Viollet B, Guigas B, Sanz Garcia N, et al. Cellular and molecular mechanisms of metformin: an overview. Clin Sci (Lond) 2012;122(6):253–70.

3. Zou MH, Kirkpatrick SS, Davis BJ, et al. Activation of the AMP-activated protein kinase by the anti-diabetic drug metformin in vivo. Role of mitochondrial reactive nitrogen species. J Biol Chem 2004;279(42):43940–51.

4. Ouyang J, Parakhia RA, Ochs RS. Metformin activates AMP kinase through inhibition of AMP deaminase. J Biol Chem 2011;286(1):1–11.

5. Myerburg MM, King JD Jr, Oyster NM, et al. AMPK agonists ameliorate sodium and fluid transport and inflammation in cystic fibrosis airway epithelial cells. Am J Respir Cell Mol Biol 2010;42(6):676–84.

6. Clark AR. MAP kinase phosphatase 1: a novel mediator of biological effects of glucocorticoids? J Endocrinol 2003;178(1):5–12.

7. Todd DC, Armstrong S, D'Silva L, et al. Effect of obesity on airway inflammation: a cross-sectional analysis of body mass index and sputum cell counts. Clin Exp Allergy 2007;37(7):1049–54.

8. McLachlan CR, Poulton R, Car G, et al. Adiposity, asthma, and airway inflammation. J Allergy Clin Immunol 2007;119(3):634–9.

9. Desai D, Newby C, Symon FA, et al. Elevated sputum interleukin-5 and submucosal eosinophilia in obese individuals with severe asthma. Am J Respir Crit Care Med 2013;188(6):657–63.

10. Calixto MC, Lintomen L, Andre DM, et al. Metformin attenuates the exacerbation of the allergic eosinophilic inflammation in high fat-diet-induced obesity in mice. PLoS One 2013;8(10):e76786.

11. Park CS, Bang BR, Kwon HS, et al. Metformin reduces airway inflammation and remodeling via activation of AMP-activated protein kinase. Biochem Pharmacol 2012;84(12):1660–70.

12. Morrow VA, Foufelle F, Connell JM, et al. Direct activation of AMP-activated protein kinase stimulates nitric-oxide synthesis in human aortic endothelial cells. J Biol Chem 2003;278(34):31629–39.

13. Davis B, Rahman A, Arner A. AMP-activated kinase relaxes agonist induced contractions in the mouse aorta via effects on PKC signaling and inhibits NO-induced relaxation. Eur J Pharmacol 2012;695(1–3):88–95.

14. Cheang WS, Tian XY, Wong WT, et al. Metformin protects endothelial function in diet-induced obese mice by inhibition of endoplasmic reticulum stress through 5' adenosine monophosphate-activated protein kinase-peroxisome proliferator-activated receptor delta pathway. Arterioscler Thromb Vasc Biol 2014;34:830–6.

15. Tabit CE, Shenouda SM, Holbrook M, et al. Protein kinase C-beta contributes to impaired endothelial insulin signaling in humans with diabetes mellitus. Circulation 2013;127(1):86–95.

16. Ahmad T, Mabalirajan U, Joseph DA, et al. Exhaled nitric oxide estimation by a simple and efficient noninvasive technique and its utility as a marker of airway inflammation in mice. J Appl Physiol (1985) 2009;107(1):295–301.

17. Morris CR, Poljakovic M, Lavrisha L, et al. Decreased arginine bioavailability and increased serum arginase activity in asthma. Am J Respir Crit Care Med 2004; 170(2):148–53.

18. Bratt JM, Williams K, Rabowsky MF, et al. Nitric oxide synthase enzymes in the airways of mice exposed to ovalbumin: NOS2 expression is NOS3 dependent. Mediators Inflamm 2010;2010. pii:321061.

19. Ten Broeke R, De Crom R, Van Haperen R, et al. Overexpression of endothelial nitric oxide synthase suppresses features of allergic asthma in mice. Respir Res 2006;7:58.

20. Yeganeh B, Wiechec E, Ande SR, et al. Targeting the mevalonate cascade as a new therapeutic approach in heart disease, cancer and pulmonary disease. Pharmacol Ther 2014;143:87–110.

21. Rikitake Y, Liao JK. Rho GTPases, statins, and nitric oxide. Circ Res 2005; 97(12):1232–5.

22. Takeda N, Kondo M, Ito S, et al. Role of RhoA inactivation in reduced cell proliferation of human airway smooth muscle by simvastatin. Am J Respir Cell Mol Biol 2006;35(6):722–9.

23. Vigano T, Hernandez A, Corsini A, et al. Mevalonate pathway and isoprenoids regulate human bronchial myocyte proliferation. Eur J Pharmacol 1995;291(2): 201–3.

24. Romero MJ, Platt DH, Tawfik HE, et al. Diabetes-induced coronary vascular dysfunction involves increased arginase activity. Circ Res 2008;102(1):95–102.

25. Romero MJ, Iddings JA, Platt DH, et al. Diabetes-induced vascular dysfunction involves arginase I. Am J Physiol Heart Circ Physiol 2012;302(1):H159–166.

26. Holowatz LA, Santhanam L, Webb A, et al. Oral atorvastatin therapy restores cutaneous microvascular function by decreasing arginase activity in hypercholesterolaemic humans. J Physiol 2011;589(Pt 8):2093–103.

27. Zeki AA, Thai P, Kenyon NJ, et al. Differential effects of simvastatin on IL-13-induced cytokine gene expression in primary mouse tracheal epithelial cells. Respir Res 2012;13:38.

28. Zeki AA, Bratt JM, Rabowsky M, et al. Simvastatin inhibits goblet cell hyperplasia and lung arginase in a mouse model of allergic asthma: a novel treatment for airway remodeling? Transl Res 2010;156(6):335–49.

29. Rossoni LV, Wareing M, Wenceslau CF, et al. Acute simvastatin increases endothelial nitric oxide synthase phosphorylation via AMP-activated protein kinase and reduces contractility of isolated rat mesenteric resistance arteries. Clin Sci (Lond) 2011;121(10):449–58.

30. Sun W, Lee TS, Zhu M, et al. Statins activate AMP-activated protein kinase in vitro and in vivo. Circulation 2006;114(24):2655–62.

31. Gillespie JG, Hardie DG. Phosphorylation and inactivation of HMG-CoA reductase at the AMP-activated protein kinase site in response to fructose treatment of isolated rat hepatocytes. FEBS Lett 1992;306(1):59–62.

32. Fisslthaler B, Fleming I, Keseru B, et al. Fluid shear stress and NO decrease the activity of the hydroxy-methylglutaryl coenzyme A reductase in endothelial cells via the AMP-activated protein kinase and FoxO1. Circ Res 2007;100(2):e12–21.

33. Chiba Y, Sato S, Misawa M. Lovastatin inhibits antigen-induced airway eosinophilia without affecting the production of inflammatory mediators in mice. Inflamm Res 2009;58(7):363–9.

34. Zeki AA, Franzi L, Last J, et al. Simvastatin inhibits airway hyperreactivity: implications for the mevalonate pathway and beyond. Am J Respir Crit Care Med 2009;180(8):731–40.

35. Ahmad T, Mabalirajan U, Sharma A, et al. Simvastatin improves epithelial dysfunction and airway hyperresponsiveness: from asymmetric dimethylarginine to asthma. Am J Respir Cell Mol Biol 2011;44(4):531–9.

36. Xu L, Dong XW, Shen LL, et al. Simvastatin delivery via inhalation attenuates airway inflammation in a murine model of asthma. Int Immunopharmacol 2012;12(4):556–64.

37. Chiba Y, Sato S, Hanazaki M, et al. Inhibition of geranylgeranyltransferase inhibits bronchial smooth muscle hyperresponsiveness in mice. Am J Physiol Lung Cell Mol Physiol 2009;297(5):L984–991.

38. Zeki AA, Oldham J, Wilson M, et al. Statin use and asthma control in patients with severe asthma. BMJ Open 2013;3(8). pii:e003314.

39. Boger RH, Mugge A, Bode-Boger SM, et al. Differential systemic and pulmonary hemodynamic effects of L-arginine in patients with coronary artery disease or primary pulmonary hypertension. Int J Clin Pharmacol Ther 1996;34(8): 323–8.

40. Dorniak-Wall T, Grivell RM, Dekker GA, et al. The role of L-arginine in the prevention and treatment of pre-eclampsia: a systematic review of randomised trials. J Hum Hypertens 2014;28(4):230–5.

41. Bednarz B, Jaxa-Chamiec T, Maciejewski P, et al. Efficacy and safety of oral l-arginine in acute myocardial infarction. Results of the multicenter, randomized, double-blind, placebo-controlled ARAMI pilot trial. Kardiol Pol 2005;62(5): 421–7.

42. Sullivan KJ, Kissoon N, Sandler E, et al. Effect of oral arginine supplementation on exhaled nitric oxide concentration in sickle cell anemia and acute chest syndrome. J Pediatr Hematol Oncol 2010;32(7):e249–258.

43. Zaobornyj T, Ghafourifar P. Strategic localization of heart mitochondrial NOS: a review of the evidence. Am J Physiol Heart Circ Physiol 2012;303(11): H1283–1293.

44. Xia Y, Dawson VL, Dawson TM, et al. Nitric oxide synthase generates superoxide and nitric oxide in arginine-depleted cells leading to peroxynitrite-mediated cellular injury. Proc Natl Acad Sci U S A 1996;93(13):6770–4.

45. Chen CA, Wang TY, Varadharaj S, et al. S-glutathionylation uncouples eNOS and regulates its cellular and vascular function. Nature 2010;468(7327):1115–8.

46. North ML, Khanna N, Marsden PA, et al. Functionally important role for arginase 1 in the airway hyperresponsiveness of asthma. Am J Physiol Lung Cell Mol Physiol 2009;296(6):L911–920.

47. Maarsingh H, Dekkers BG, Zuidhof AB, et al. Increased arginase activity contributes to airway remodelling in chronic allergic asthma. Eur Respir J 2011; 38(2):318–28.

48. Meurs H, McKay S, Maarsingh H, et al. Increased arginase activity underlies allergen-induced deficiency of cNOS-derived nitric oxide and airway hyperresponsiveness. Br J Pharmacol 2002;136(3):391–8.

49. Takahashi N, Ogino K, Takemoto K, et al. Direct inhibition of arginase attenuated airway allergic reactions and inflammation in a Dermatophagoides farinae-induced NC/Nga mouse model. Am J Physiol Lung Cell Mol Physiol 2010; 299(1):L17–24.

50. Bratt JM, Franzi LM, Linderholm AL, et al. Arginase inhibition in airways from normal and nitric oxide synthase 2-knockout mice exposed to ovalbumin. Toxicol Appl Pharmacol 2010;242(1):1–8.

51. Mabalirajan U, Ahmad T, Leishangthem GD, et al. Beneficial effects of high dose of L-arginine on airway hyperresponsiveness and airway inflammation in a murine model of asthma. J Allergy Clin Immunol 2010;125(3):626–35.

52. Kim OY, Lee SM, Chung JH, et al. Arginase I and the very low-density lipoprotein receptor are associated with phenotypic biomarkers for obesity. Nutrition 2012; 28(6):635–9.

53. Giri H, Muthuramu I, Dhar M, et al. Protein tyrosine phosphatase SHP2 mediates chronic insulin-induced endothelial inflammation. Arterioscler Thromb Vasc Biol 2012;32(8):1943–50.

54. Johnson FK, Johnson RA, Peyton KJ, et al. Arginase promotes skeletal muscle arteriolar endothelial dysfunction in diabetic rats. Front Immunol 2013;4:119.

55. Holguin F, Comhair SA, Hazen SL, et al. An association between L-arginine/asymmetric dimethyl arginine balance, obesity, and the age of asthma onset phenotype. Am J Respir Crit Care Med 2013;187(2):153–9.

56. Bedford MT, Richard S. Arginine methylation an emerging regulator of protein function. Mol Cell 2005;18(3):263–72.

57. Bulau P, Zakrzewicz D, Kitowska K, et al. Analysis of methylarginine metabolism in the cardiovascular system identifies the lung as a major source of ADMA. Am J Physiol Lung Cell Mol Physiol 2007;292(1):L18–24.

58. Rawal N, Rajpurohit R, Lischwe MA, et al. Structural specificity of substrate for S-adenosylmethionine:protein arginine N-methyltransferases. Biochim Biophys Acta 1995;1248(1):11–8.

59. Cantoni GL. Biological methylation: selected aspects. Annu Rev Biochem 1975; 44:435–51.

60. MacAllister RJ, Fickling SA, Whitley GS, et al. Metabolism of methylarginines by human vasculature; implications for the regulation of nitric oxide synthesis. Br J Pharmacol 1994;112(1):43–8.

61. Scott JA, North ML, Rafii M, et al. Asymmetric dimethylarginine is increased in asthma. Am J Respir Crit Care Med 2011;184(7):779–85.

62. Kato GJ, Wang Z, Machado RF, et al. Endogenous nitric oxide synthase inhibitors in sickle cell disease: abnormal levels and correlations with pulmonary hypertension, desaturation, haemolysis, organ dysfunction and death. Br J Haematol 2009;145(4):506–13.

63. Abbasi F, Asagmi T, Cooke JP, et al. Plasma concentrations of asymmetric dimethylarginine are increased in patients with type 2 diabetes mellitus. Am J Cardiol 2001;88(10):1201–3.

64. Eid HM, Arnesen H, Hjerkinn EM, et al. Relationship between obesity, smoking, and the endogenous nitric oxide synthase inhibitor, asymmetric dimethylarginine. Metabolism 2004;53(12):1574–9.

65. Stuhlinger MC, Abbasi F, Chu JW, et al. Relationship between insulin resistance and an endogenous nitric oxide synthase inhibitor. JAMA 2002;287(11):1420–6.

66. Sydow K, Mondon CE, Cooke JP. Insulin resistance: potential role of the endogenous nitric oxide synthase inhibitor ADMA. Vasc Med 2005;10(Suppl 1): S35–43.

67. Ahmad T, Mabalirajan U, Ghosh B, et al. Altered asymmetric dimethyl arginine metabolism in allergically inflamed mouse lungs. Am J Respir Cell Mol Biol 2010;42(1):3–8.

68. Kinker KG, Gibson AM, Bass SA, et al. Overexpression of dimethylarginine dimethylaminohydrolase 1 attenuates airway inflammation in a mouse model of asthma. PLoS One 2014;9(1):e85148.

69. Pullamsetti SS, Savai R, Schaefer MB, et al. cAMP phosphodiesterase inhibitors increases nitric oxide production by modulating dimethylarginine dimethylaminohydrolases. Circulation 2011;123(11):1194–204.

70. Hwang TL, Tang MC, Kuo LM, et al. YC-1 potentiates cAMP-induced CREB activation and nitric oxide production in alveolar macrophages. Toxicol Appl Pharmacol 2012;260(2):193–200.

71. Qiao J, Huang F, Lum H. PKA inhibits RhoA activation: a protection mechanism against endothelial barrier dysfunction. Am J Physiol Lung Cell Mol Physiol 2003;284(6):L972–980.

72. Ming XF, Barandier C, Viswambharan H, et al. Thrombin stimulates human endothelial arginase enzymatic activity via RhoA/ROCK pathway: implications for atherosclerotic endothelial dysfunction. Circulation 2004;110(24):3708–14.

73. Belleguic C, Corbel M, Germain N, et al. Reduction of matrix metalloproteinase-9 activity by the selective phosphodiesterase 4 inhibitor, RP 73-401 in sensitized mice. Eur J Pharmacol 2000;404(3):369–73.

74. Kumar RK, Herbert C, Thomas PS, et al. Inhibition of inflammation and remodeling by roflumilast and dexamethasone in murine chronic asthma. J Pharmacol Exp Ther 2003;307(1):349–55.

75. Allen S, Britton JR, Leonardi-Bee JA. Association between antioxidant vitamins and asthma outcome measures: systematic review and meta-analysis. Thorax 2009;64(7):610–9.

76. Ahmad SM, Haskell MJ, Raqib R, et al. Vitamin A status is associated with T-cell responses in Bangladeshi men. Br J Nutr 2009;102(6):797–802.

77. Ross AC. Vitamin A and retinoic acid in T cell-related immunity. Am J Clin Nutr 2012;96(5):1166S–72S.

78. Finklea JD, Grossmann RE, Tangpricha V. Vitamin D and chronic lung disease: a review of molecular mechanisms and clinical studies. Adv Nutr 2011;2(3):244–53.

79. Paul G, Brehm JM, Alcorn JF, et al. Vitamin D and asthma. Am J Respir Crit Care Med 2012;185(2):124–32.

80. Pathak K, Soares MJ, Calton EK, et al. Vitamin D supplementation and body weight status: a systematic review and meta-analysis of randomized controlled trials. Obes Rev 2014;15:528–37.

81. Milan SJ, Hart A, Wilkinson M. Vitamin C for asthma and exercise-induced bronchoconstriction. Cochrane Database Syst Rev 2013;(10):CD010391.

82. Trenga CA, Koenig JQ, Williams PV. Dietary antioxidants and ozone-induced bronchial hyperresponsiveness in adults with asthma. Arch Environ Health 2001;56(3):242–9.

83. Keaney JF Jr, Gaziano JM, Xu A, et al. Dietary antioxidants preserve endothelium-dependent vessel relaxation in cholesterol-fed rabbits. Proc Natl Acad Sci U S A 1993;90(24):11880–4.

84. Schuster GU, Kenyon NJ, Stephensen CB. Asthma. In: Caballero B, editor. Encyclopedia of human nutrition, vol. 1, 3rd edition. Elsevier, Ltd; 2013. p. 122–8.

85. Nakamura T, Azuma A, Kuribayashi T, et al. Serum fatty acid levels, dietary style and coronary heart disease in three neighbouring areas in Japan: the Kumihama study. Br J Nutr 2003;89(2):267–72.

86. Bjerregaard P, Pedersen HS, Mulvad G. The associations of a marine diet with plasma lipids, blood glucose, blood pressure and obesity among the inuit in Greenland. Eur J Clin Nutr 2000;54(9):732–7.

87. Schmitz G, Ecker J. The opposing effects of n−3 and n−6 fatty acids. Prog Lipid Res 2008;47(2):147–55.

88. Serhan CN, Chiang N, Van Dyke TE. Resolving inflammation: dual anti-inflammatory and pro-resolution lipid mediators. Nat Rev Immunol 2008;8(5):349–61.

Nutritional Influences on Epigenetic Programming
Asthma, Allergy, and Obesity

Debra J. Palmer, PhD[a,b,*], Rae-Chi Huang, MD, PhD[b,c], Jeffrey M. Craig, PhD[d], Susan L. Prescott, MD, PhD[a,b,c]

KEYWORDS

- Nutrition • Early life • Epigenetic regulation • Asthma • Allergy • Obesity

KEY POINTS

- Maternal and infant nutrition play a critical role in determining the subsequent risk of asthma, allergic diseases, and obesity.
- Modern dietary patterns (including less consumption of vegetables, legumes, and fish) result in reduced antiinflammatory nutrient intakes, in particular prebiotics, antioxidants, and omega-3 long-chain fatty acids.
- Antiinflammatory nutrients modulate the developmental programming of metabolic and immune pathways, and increase the risk of the chronic inflammation and immune dysregulation seen in association with asthma, allergic diseases, and obesity.
- Epigenetics is providing substantial advances in understanding how early-life nutritional exposures can affect disease development.

INTRODUCTION

Nutrition in early life, especially from conception until 2 years of age (the first 1000 days), has a major influence on later predisposition to many noncommunicable diseases (NCDs), including cardiovascular, metabolic, and allergic diseases. Barker[1] laid the core foundations by showing the relationships between early-life conditions (particularly nutritional status) and the subsequent risk of cardiovascular and

The authors have nothing to disclose.

[a] School of Paediatrics and Child Health, University of Western Australia (M561), Roberts Road, Subiaco, Western Australia 6008, Australia; [b] Members of 'In-FLAME' the International Inflammation Network, World Universities Network (WUN); [c] Telethon KIDS Institute, University of Western Australia, Roberts Road, Subiaco, Western Australia 6008, Australia; [d] Department of Paediatrics, University of Melbourne and Early Life Epigenetics Group, Murdoch Children's Research Institute, Royal Children's Hospital, Flemington Road, Parkville, Victoria 3052, Australia

* Corresponding author. School of Paediatrics and Child Health, University of Western Australia (M561), Roberts Road, Subiaco, Western Australia 6008, Australia.
E-mail address: debbie.palmer@uwa.edu.au

Immunol Allergy Clin N Am 34 (2014) 825–837
http://dx.doi.org/10.1016/j.iac.2014.07.003
0889-8561/14/$ – see front matter
immunology.theclinics.com

metabolic diseases many decades later. This paradigm of developmental programming, now known as developmental origins of health and disease (DOHaD), has been extended to many other organ systems through a large range of cohort studies, mechanistic studies, and animal models. More recently, these have revealed that one of the main mechanisms through which nutrition can influence these long-term health outcomes is via modulation of epigenetic programming. Epigenetic mechanisms can be broadly defined as a network of biological processes that regulate the expression of genes to produce mitotically heritable changes in cellular function without changes in the underlying DNA sequence.[2] These processes include DNA methylation, post-translational modification to histone tails, and regulation through noncoding RNAs. This knowledge has provided new insights into how subsequent patterns of gene expression can be changed by a range of early nutritional and environmental factors to alter the risk of both early-onset and late-onset NCDs, and has become the cornerstone of DOHaD research.[3]

New so-called modern epidemics such as allergic disease, which is an early-onset NCD, provide evidence that the immune system is specifically vulnerable to recent environmental, diet, and lifestyle changes.[4] Over the past 2 decades there has been a dramatic increase in the incidence of allergic disease, especially food allergy, in the first few years of life.[5,6] Over the same period there has been a parallel increase in obesity,[7,8] and there have been suggestions that allergic disease and obesity may be associated.[9] It is also increasingly clear that both immune and metabolic programming are under epigenetic regulation. This article discusses recent evidence focusing on the influence of nutrition on metabolic and immune pathways that are likely to underpin the increasing rates of allergy, obesity, and other inflammatory diseases, with a particular focus on the epigenetic mechanisms.

EPIGENETICS, OBESITY, AND ASTHMA

Epigenetics has provided a substantial advance in understanding of how the early environment, including early-life nutritional exposures, can have effects on disease propensity much later in life. There are now many examples of how nutritional exposures in utero can induce differential effects on epigenetic machinery. These alterations in epigenetic marks are associated with either enhanced or suppressed gene expression with an altered phenotype depending on the nature of the affected biological pathways.[2]

In humans, Fryer and colleagues[10] analyzed the cytosine-guanine dinucleotide (CpG) dinucleotide methylation in 12 cord blood samples using high-resolution genomewide methylation profiling, and levels of plasma homocysteine, a metabolite of folate, correlated with infant DNA methylation patterns and birth weight. In addition, it has been shown that periconceptional maternal folic acid supplementation can lead to a higher methylation level of the differentially methylated region in the IGF2 gene in children.[11] In this study, DNA methylation was inversely correlated with birth weight. IGF2 is an important regulator of fetal growth that mediates its effects through the IGF1 receptor (IGF1R), and observed differential methylation patterns in IGF2 and IGF1R in relation to maternal folic acid intake suggest that maternal folic acid intake influences fetal growth and metabolism.

Obesity and Epigenetics

In the context of the development of obesity, experimental evidence shows a causative link between early-life nutritional challenges and the risk of subsequent obesity and metabolic disease.[12–14] In animal models, exposure to maternal obesity and high-fat diets influences the risk of obesity in the offspring. Vucetic and colleagues[15] showed that obese mothers fed a high-fat diet had offspring with epigenetic changes in key genes controlling appetite and metabolism. Borengasser and colleagues[16] recently found hepatic mRNA expression of circadian (*CLOCK, BMAL1, REV-ERBa, CRY, PER*) and metabolic (*PPARa, SIRT1*) genes were strongly suppressed in offspring exposed to both maternal obesity and a high-fat diet.

Animal studies have also determined that early-life exposure to bisphenol A (BPA), a high-production-volume chemical used in the manufacture of polycarbonate plastic, can change offspring phenotype by stably altering the epigenome. However, this effect can be counteracted by maternal dietary supplements. Using an agouti mouse model, Dolinoy and colleagues[17] showed that in utero exposure to BPA is associated with higher body weight by decreasing CpG methylation. However maternal dietary supplementation, with either methyl donors like folic acid[17] or genistein (the major phytoestrogen in soy),[18] negated the DNA hypomethylating effect of BPA.

Human evidence of altered DNA methylation leading to fetal programming of obesity was first seen at the *IGF2/H19* locus. During the Dutch Hunger Winter in the 1940s, offspring were exposed to maternal famine early in gestation. Sixty years later, these offspring had decreased methylation in a region controlling expression within the *IGF2* locus[19] accompanied by increased obesity.[20] Periconceptional folate supplementation has been associated with altered DNA methylation in the imprinting control region of *IGF2/H19*[21] and overweight status at 12 months of age.[22] DNA methylation at the *IGF2/H19* imprinting control region has also been positively associated with subscapular, suprailiac, abdominal, and triceps skin fold thickness and subcutaneous fat thickness in adolescents.[23]

Differential methylation in other loci in humans has also been associated with obesity. Methylation of specific CpGs within the promoter of the retinoid X receptor alpha (*RXRA*) gene in umbilical cord tissue at birth is associated with childhood fat mass[12] and neonatal epigenetic marks and sex of the infant explained more than 25% of the variance in childhood obesity.[12] Another example is the finding that DNA methylation in the peroxisomal proliferator gamma coactivator 1-alpha promoter in blood predicted adiposity up to 14 years of age independently of sex, age, pubertal timing, and physical activity.[24]

Asthma and Epigenetics

Although a family history of asthma and allergic disease is a strong predictor of asthma development, there seem to be many influential environmental, lifestyle, and dietary factors that modify the inheritable risk. In particular, maternal exposure to cigarette smoke and air pollution during pregnancy are known to increase the risk,[25,26] whereas a maternal diet during pregnancy high in fish, legumes, and vegetables decreases the risk.[27]

Epigenetic changes are likely to improve future understanding of, and strategies for, asthma prevention. Using an adult cohort of monozygotic twins discordant for asthma, Runyon and colleagues[28] showed increased levels of CpG methylation within the FOXP3 locus, decreased FOXP3 protein expression, and impaired regulatory T-cell function. In parallel, Runyon and colleagues[28] also showed increased methylation of the *IFNG* locus, decreased *IFNG* expression, and reduced effector T-cell function in the asthmatic twin compared with the nonasthmatic twin. Patil and colleagues[29] investigated DNA methylation of the interleukin (IL)-13 gene and found interactions with asthma-related lung function. The findings from Soto-Ramirez and colleagues[30] also suggest that DNA methylation modulates the risk of asthma in association with genetic variants in the IL-4R gene.

Further to this, a recent pilot study (n = 32)[31] found differences in DNA methylation between children with obesity-associated asthma compared with children with obesity but without asthma, nonobese asthmatic children, and healthy normal-weight controls. This study investigated epigenomewide DNA methylation in peripheral blood mononuclear cells (PBMCs) collected from preadolescent children. PBMCs from 8 obese asthmatic children had decreased promoter methylation of CCL5, IL2RA, and TBX21 genes, which encode proteins linked to Th1 polarization, innate immune, and nonatopic patterns of inflammation. This study also found that PBMCs from obese asthmatic children had increased promoter methylation of FCER2 and TGFB1. Together, these differences in methylation profiles were associated with T-cell differentiation and increased macrophage activation, which have previously been linked to the pathophysiology of obesity-associated asthma.[32,33] Future studies further examining the potential dietary and/or lifestyle factors that may have preceded these DNA methylation effects will be of key importance.

MULTIPLE EPIGENETIC EFFECTS OF NUTRITIONAL EXPOSURES

Methyl donors such as folate, methionine, and choline derived from the diet are of much interest because of their role in DNA methylation through 1-carbon metabolism.[34] Furthermore, a range of other nutritional factors, including vitamin D,[35] antioxidants (such as selenium; zinc; and vitamins A, C, and E),[36,37] long-chain polyunsaturated fatty acids (LCPUFAs),[38] and short-chain fatty acids (SCFAs),[39] also seem to modulate gene expression through epigenetic effects. Diet-induced changes in the microbiome[40] and even food contaminants such as bisphenol A[41,42] can also induce epigenetic changes in genes in metabolic and/or immune networks to influence the risk of disease. Although many of these effects have been shown in animal models, more evidence in humans is greatly needed.

FOLATE (FOLIC ACID) AND DNA METHYLATION

In the early 1990s, randomized controlled trials (RCTs)[43,44] found that folic acid supplementation in the periconceptional period significantly reduced the risk of occurrence of neural tube defects (NTDs). Over the past 20 years, folic acid supplementation of 400 μg/day at least 1 month before and 3 months after conception has been recommended, in addition to consuming folate from foods in a varied diet. The widespread use of maternal folate supplementation in the periconceptional period has been effective at reducing the risk of NTDs. However, long-term effects of maternal folate supplementation, particularly when continued at high doses after the window of risk for NTDs has passed (beyond 3 months after conception), on other health outcomes are less clear.

In a highly cited murine study, Hollingsworth and colleagues[45] showed that maternal folic acid supplementation modifies the expression of immune genes in the offspring through changes in DNA methylation, with associated development of an allergic phenotype; specifically, an enhanced severity of allergic airway disease in mice offspring. Furthermore, evidence from an Australian human prospective birth cohort study[46] shows that folic acid taken in supplement form in late pregnancy was associated with an increased risk of childhood asthma at 3.5 years. Another Australian study found that infants exposed in utero to more than 500 μg/day of maternal folic acid supplementation during late pregnancy (third trimester) were more likely to develop eczema during infancy.[47] A recent meta-analysis[48] (cohort and case-control studies; no RCTs), found no evidence of an association between maternal folic acid supplementation use in the periconceptional period (before and during the first trimester of pregnancy) and asthma during childhood (0–8 years) in the offspring. Thus it seems that the timing of exposure to folate supplementation in utero may be critical with regard to childhood allergic disease outcomes.

An interesting recent study using Wistar rats[49] also provides new evidence on metabolic effects related to the timing and duration of a high-folate diet in early life. This study found improved metabolic outcomes in pups exposed to a high-folate diet both in utero as well as a high-folate postnatal diet, compared with a normal postnatal diet. These improved metabolic outcomes included lower food intake, reduced weight gain, and improved glucose response to both a glucose load and an insulin load. This new animal study evidence supports the hypothesis that folate can modify hypothalamic feeding pathways in rat offspring, possibly because of epigenetic alterations in DNA methylation. The results from this study suggest that in utero programming can be further modified by early postnatal diets. Further research in this field is needed to better define the effects of timing and duration of folate supplementation during early life on early and later health outcomes. More studies, specifically epigenome-wide association studies, are also needed to explore the wider epigenetic effects of folic acid supplementation.

BEYOND FOLATE: EPIGENETICS AND OTHER NUTRIENTS

In recent years, several other key nutrients, including antioxidants, vitamin D, LCPUFAs, and SCFAs, have been linked to multiple health outcomes, including asthma and allergic diseases, as well as obesity. Research is currently underway investigating possible epigenetic effects of changing the dietary intake of these nutrients, especially in the maternal diet during pregnancy and the early postnatal period.

Antioxidants

In vitro human studies have shown that antioxidants (such as selenium; zinc; vitamins A, C, and E) favorably alter the redox status of cells by enhancing IL-12 production by antigen-presenting cells to promote Th1 differentiation,[50] although it is not clear whether this can be extrapolated to the in vivo setting. Observational studies suggest that higher dietary intakes of antioxidant-rich foods (such as fresh fruits and vegetables) or higher antioxidant levels measured in pregnancy[51,52] and early childhood[53,54] may reduce the risk of wheezing, asthma, and/or eczema. As yet there are no intervention studies in early life to directly examine potential preventive effects. In part, this has been because there are 2 contrary hypotheses around the role of dietary antioxidant intake and immune outcomes. Although antioxidants have been suggested to protect against allergic disease, there is also an alternative hypothesis that proposes a theoretic concern that antioxidant supplementation could increase the probability of Th2 differentiation (by inhibiting oxidative stress) and favor the development of asthma and allergic disease.[55] As for other nutrients, the dose, timing, and duration in early life of antioxidant exposures are likely to be critical.

Long Chain Polyunsaturated Fatty Acids

Dietary omega-3 LCPUFAs have been shown to have multisystem antiinflammatory benefits on both immune and metabolic outcomes. Several RCTs investigating maternal fish oil supplementation during pregnancy have found beneficial effects on immunomodulatory effects in cord blood,[56–58] with reduced allergen sensitization and allergic disease outcomes in the offspring.[57,59–61] Maternal fish oil supplementation in pregnancy lowers neonatal oxidative stress[56] and neutrophil production of leukotriene B4, which correlated with reduced toll-like receptor 4 (TLR 4) mediated inflammatory responses.[58] Other studies have also found benefits for metabolic programming[62] and reducing cardiovascular risk,[63,64] with higher dietary intakes of omega-3 LCPUFAs in early life.

Recent studies in mice and rats[38,65] have found some evidence that maternal fat intake (both quantity and fatty acid composition) during pregnancy and lactation can cause changes in the epigenetic regulation of the offspring. Niculescu and colleagues[65] showed higher DNA methylation of the *Fads2* promoter after mice were given a postnatal flaxseed oil containing 50% alpha-linolenic acid (mothers or pups). Hoile and colleagues[38] found decreased *Fads2* mRNA expression associated with increased methylation of CpG loci in the *Fads2* promoter in the rat offspring after increasing maternal dietary fat content. This effect on epigenetic regulation was observed to continue into adulthood. Human studies are needed and currently this field of research is still in its infancy, but it will be important to interpret some of the findings of human RCTs investigating the role of omega-3 LCPUFA supplementation during pregnancy and early life on multiple health outcomes.

Vitamin D

A particular challenge will be investigating the possible role of vitamin D in epigenetic regulation. It has been estimated that around 2000 genes may be directly or indirectly regulated by various vitamin D metabolites, and possible epigenetic effects are currently thought to be involved with histone modifications, especially acetylation, and mediated by the nuclear vitamin D receptor.[66] Vitamin D status is influenced by environmental factors through sunlight exposure as well as dietary sources, through foods naturally rich in vitamin D (including fatty fish and cod liver oil), foods fortified with vitamin D in some countries (including milk and margarine), as well as the use of oral vitamin D supplementation in some populations.[66] It will be important to study the possible effects of changes to vitamin D status during early life. In particular, will there be epigenetic regulation effects in which a child experiences an in utero environment high in vitamin D from maternal oral vitamin D supplementation during pregnancy, but low vitamin D status during infancy? In the future, some of the current controversies, especially surrounding the effects of vitamin D status or use of supplementation in early life on allergic disease development, may be explained by epigenetic regulation effects.

GUT MICROBIOTA BIODIVERSITY AND SHORT-CHAIN FATTY ACIDS

Modern diets typically contain more processed, low-fiber foods than more traditional diets.[67,68] In particular, diets are generally containing less fruit, vegetables, unprocessed grains, nuts, and seeds. This dietary pattern with reduced fiber content is associated with changes in gut microbiota biodiversity, which is another common risk factor now strongly linked with both allergy and obesity.[40] The gut microbiota and its collective genetic material (the microbiome) have emerged as important factors in normal immune development. Although the original focus of the so-called hygiene hypothesis was on declining infectious exposures, disruption of the nonpathogenic commensal gut microbiota is now recognized as a potentially greater risk for early immune and metabolic dysregulation, and is implicated in the increasing risk of obesity and many associated inflammatory NCDs.[40] Changing composition of gut microflora has been linked to associated inflammation and disruptions in gut homeostasis and immune maturation, with altered gut barrier function, increased systemic endotoxin, and low-grade TLR-mediated systemic inflammation with increased C-reactive protein, IL-1β, tumor necrosis factor, and IL-6.[69–71]

Animal models provide evidence that the gut microbiota modulate immune programming, and that manipulation of the microbiome can prevent not only allergic disease[72,73] but also the risk of obesity, cardiovascular disease, and metabolic disease through well-described metabolic effects.[74] The use of soluble prebiotic fiber (oligosaccharides) has similarly been shown to have beneficial effects on both immune[75] and metabolic homeostasis.[76] Prebiotic fermentation products, SCFAs, have antiinflammatory effects[77] that promote intestinal integrity and reduce systemic endotoxin and antigenic load in experimental models. SCFAs play a critical role in local and systemic metabolic function and stimulate regulatory immune responses.[78] There is newly emerging evidence of effects of SCFA-producing bacteria on epigenetic regulation of metabolic genes, notably free fatty acid receptor in type 2 diabetes and obesity.[39] Our collaborators are also currently examining the epigenetic effects of SCFAs on immune genes.

The Importance of Antenatal Nutrition and Maternal Biodiversity

Most studies investigating the early immune-modulatory mechanisms have focused on postnatal microbial diversity.[79,80] However, it is increasingly clear that the maternal environment, nutrition, and gut biodiversity during pregnancy are also important in early immune programming.[40,81] We have shown emergent differences in immune function at birth in newborns destined to develop allergy,[82,83] indicating that the scene is set to some extent by birth. Experimental animal models show that maternal treatment with commensal bacteria such as *Lactobacillus rhamnosus*[84] or other apathogenic bacteria such as *Acinetobacter lwoffii*[85] during pregnancy attenuate allergic sensitization and inflammation in the offspring. These effects are mediated by activation of maternal innate immune pathways, namely TLR signaling,[85] with associated epigenetic effects in immune genes (*IFNG*) in the newborn offspring.[86] This finding is consistent with human evidence that maternal probiotics in late pregnancy significantly modulate the expression of TLR-related genes both in placenta and the fetal gut.[87]

Studies of specific prebiotic oligosaccharides in pregnancy are still limited. In animal models prebiotics alter colonization and metabolic homeostasis,[88] and reduce eczemalike inflammation in offspring.[89] To our knowledge, the only human RCT to use prebiotics in pregnancy was too small (n = 48) to reliably assess immune effects on the fetus or clinical effects, but did achieve favorable changes in maternal gut microbiota.[90] Larger human trials of prebiotics in pregnancy are needed to examine these effects further, including the interplay between metabolic and immune effects.

IMPORTANCE OF A WHOLE DIETARY COMPOSITION APPROACH RATHER THAN INDIVIDUAL NUTRIENTS

Research in this topic is not straightforward and inconsistencies in the human evidence base to date are likely to reflect the inherent complexity of each individual's diet, difficulty in accurately measuring it, and interplay with many other segregating environmental and lifestyle factors. Clinicians must not just consider or focus too heavily on 1 or 2 foods or nutrients, but should remember that the total diet and lifestyle combination is what is most important. For example, dietary patterns such as a Mediterranean diet have been repeatedly shown in many studies over the past decade (as reviewed in Ref.[91]) to have a protective effect against the development and progression of NCDs, including obesity. The Mediterranean diet describes the common foods and resulting dietary intake pattern that was characteristic of several countries in the Mediterranean Basin geographic region during the early 1960s.[92] The Mediterranean diet during pregnancy, in particular higher consumption of vegetables, legumes, and fish, has also been associated with protection from childhood

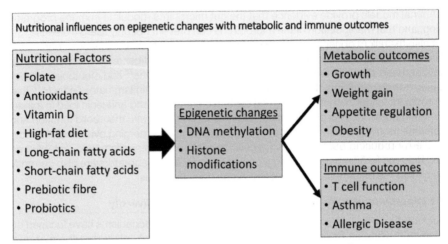

Fig. 1. Nutritional influences on epigenetic changes with metabolic and immune outcomes.

wheeze and atopy.[27] Given the evidence presented in this article, vegetables, legumes, and fish in particular are consistently shown to be beneficial dietary components, because they are good sources of many antioxidants, soluble prebiotic fiber, and omega-3 LCPUFAs. However, modern diets tend to be much lower in fish, vegetables, and legumes compared with more traditional diets.[67,68] Encouraging a healthy balanced diet, including fish, vegetables, and legumes, especially in early life (the first 1000 days) seems an obvious and logical approach to reducing the risk of asthma, allergic diseases, and obesity. However, reversing current modern dietary habits, with their increased reliance on processed and convenience foods and often with low-fiber and poor nutritional quality, is a major challenge.

SUMMARY

It is now apparent that many NCDs, including asthma and obesity, share the same common early-life nutritional risk factors. Moreover, most of the modern dietary risk factors modulate developmental programming of metabolic and immune pathways to increase the risk of the chronic inflammation and immune dysregulation seen in association with many NCDs. Changing modern dietary intakes and resulting nutritional effects on these pathways provide an obvious common element contributing to the risk and prevention of these conditions, which underscores the need to take a whole-diet approach to overcoming the increasing burden of many NCDs (**Fig. 1**).

There is no longer any doubt that maternal and infant nutrition play critical roles in determining the subsequent risk of asthma, allergic diseases, and obesity. The increasing reliance on dietary supplementation and fortification of foods (eg, with folate) may be causing more harm than benefit. Effective strategies are needed to increase dietary intakes of particular foods (eg, fish, vegetables, and legumes) and nutrients (eg, antioxidants, LCPUFAs, and SCFAs) that have many properties that protect against certain NCDs. Further research on changing nutritional intakes and epigenetic consequences will improve the evidence base.

REFERENCES

1. Barker DJ. In utero programming of chronic disease. Clin Sci 1998;95(2): 115–28.

2. Waterland RA, Michels KB. Epigenetic epidemiology of the developmental origins hypothesis. Annu Rev Nutr 2007;27:363–88.
3. Gluckman PD, Hanson MA, Mitchell MD. Developmental origins of health and disease: reducing the burden of chronic disease in the next generation. Genome Med 2010;2(2):14.
4. Prescott SL. Early-life environmental determinants of allergic diseases and the wider pandemic of inflammatory noncommunicable diseases. J Allergy Clin Immunol 2013;131(1):23–30.
5. Mullins RJ. Paediatric food allergy trends in a community-based specialist allergy practice, 1995-2006. Med J Aust 2007;186(12):618–21.
6. Prescott S, Allen KJ. Food allergy: riding the second wave of the allergy epidemic. Pediatr Allergy Immunol 2011;22(2):155–60.
7. Aekplakorn W, Inthawong R, Kessomboon P, et al. Prevalence and trends of obesity and association with socioeconomic status in Thai adults: National Health Examination Surveys, 1991-2009. J Obes 2014;2014:410259.
8. Skinner AC, Skelton JA. Prevalence and trends in obesity and severe obesity among children in the United States, 1999-2012. JAMA Pediatr 2014;168(6):561–6.
9. Visness CM, London SJ, Daniels JL, et al. Association of obesity with IgE levels and allergy symptoms in children and adolescents: results from the National Health And Nutrition Examination Survey 2005-2006. J Allergy Clin Immunol 2009;123(5):1163–9, 1169.e1–4.
10. Fryer AA, Emes RD, Ismail KM, et al. Quantitative, high-resolution epigenetic profiling of CpG loci identifies associations with cord blood plasma homocysteine and birth weight in humans. Epigenetics 2011;6(1):86–94.
11. Steegers-Theunissen RP, Obermann-Borst SA, Kremer D, et al. Periconceptional maternal folic acid use of 400 μg per day is related to increased methylation of the IGF2 gene in the very young child. PloS One 2009;4(11):e7845.
12. Godfrey KM, Sheppard A, Gluckman PD, et al. Epigenetic gene promoter methylation at birth is associated with child's later adiposity. Diabetes 2011;60(5):1528–34.
13. Lillycrop KA, Rodford J, Garratt ES, et al. Maternal protein restriction with or without folic acid supplementation during pregnancy alters the hepatic transcriptome in adult male rats. Br J Nutr 2010;103(12):1711–9.
14. Lillycrop KA, Slater-Jefferies JL, Hanson MA, et al. Induction of altered epigenetic regulation of the hepatic glucocorticoid receptor in the offspring of rats fed a protein-restricted diet during pregnancy suggests that reduced DNA methyltransferase-1 expression is involved in impaired DNA methylation and changes in histone modifications. Br J Nutr 2007;97(6):1064–73.
15. Vucetic Z, Kimmel J, Totoki K, et al. Maternal high-fat diet alters methylation and gene expression of dopamine and opioid-related genes. Endocrinology 2010;151(10):4756–64.
16. Borengasser SJ, Kang P, Faske J, et al. High fat diet and in utero exposure to maternal obesity disrupts circadian rhythm and leads to metabolic programming of liver in rat offspring. PloS One 2014;9(1):e84209.
17. Dolinoy DC, Huang D, Jirtle RL. Maternal nutrient supplementation counteracts bisphenol A-induced DNA hypomethylation in early development. Proc Natl Acad Sci U S A 2007;104(32):13056–61.
18. Dolinoy DC, Weidman JR, Waterland RA, et al. Maternal genistein alters coat color and protects Avy mouse offspring from obesity by modifying the fetal epigenome. Environ Health Perspect 2006;114(4):567–72.

19. Heijmans BT, Tobi EW, Stein AD, et al. Persistent epigenetic differences associated with prenatal exposure to famine in humans. Proc Natl Acad Sci U S A 2008;105(44):17046–9.

20. Ravelli AC, van Der Meulen JH, Osmond C, et al. Obesity at the age of 50 y in men and women exposed to famine prenatally. Am J Clin Nutr 1999;70(5):811–6.

21. Hoyo C, Murtha AP, Schildkraut JM, et al. Methylation variation at IGF2 differentially methylated regions and maternal folic acid use before and during pregnancy. Epigenetics 2011;6(7):928–36.

22. Perkins E, Murphy SK, Murtha AP, et al. Insulin-like growth factor 2/H19 methylation at birth and risk of overweight and obesity in children. J Pediatr 2012;161(1):31–9.

23. Huang RC, Galati JC, Burrows S, et al. DNA methylation of the IGF2/H19 imprinting control region and adiposity distribution in young adults. Clin Epigenetics 2012;4(1):21.

24. Clarke-Harris R, Wilkin TJ, Hosking J, et al. Peroxisomal proliferator activated receptor-gamma-co-activator-1alpha promoter methylation in blood at 5-7 years predicts adiposity from 9 to 14 years (EarlyBird 50). Diabetes 2014;63(7):2528–37.

25. Clark NA, Demers PA, Karr CJ, et al. Effect of early life exposure to air pollution on development of childhood asthma. Environ Health Perspect 2010;118(2):284–90.

26. Hylkema MN, Blacquiere MJ. Intrauterine effects of maternal smoking on sensitization, asthma, and chronic obstructive pulmonary disease. Proc Am Thorac Soc 2009;6(8):660–2.

27. Chatzi L, Torrent M, Romieu I, et al. Mediterranean diet in pregnancy is protective for wheeze and atopy in childhood. Thorax 2008;63(6):507–13.

28. Runyon RS, Cachola LM, Rajeshuni N, et al. Asthma discordance in twins is linked to epigenetic modifications of T cells. PloS One 2012;7(11):e48796.

29. Patil VK, Holloway JW, Zhang H, et al. Interaction of prenatal maternal smoking, interleukin 13 genetic variants and DNA methylation influencing airflow and airway reactivity. Clin Epigenetics 2013;5(1):22.

30. Soto-Ramirez N, Arshad SH, Holloway JW, et al. The interaction of genetic variants and DNA methylation of the interleukin-4 receptor gene increase the risk of asthma at age 18 years. Clin Epigenetics 2013;5(1):1.

31. Rastogi D, Suzuki M, Greally JM. Differential epigenome-wide DNA methylation patterns in childhood obesity-associated asthma. Sci Rep 2013;3:2164.

32. Dixon AE, Johnson SE, Griffes LV, et al. Relationship of adipokines with immune response and lung function in obese asthmatic and non-asthmatic women. J Asthma 2011;48(8):811–7.

33. Lugogo NL, Hollingsworth JW, Howell DL, et al. Alveolar macrophages from overweight/obese subjects with asthma demonstrate a proinflammatory phenotype. Am J Respir Crit Care Med 2012;186(5):404–11.

34. Craig JM, Joo JH, Novakovic B, et al. Epigenetic regulation of pregnancy outcome. In: Vaillancourt C, Lafond J, editors. Pregnancy disorders and perinatal outcomes. Sharjah: Bentham Books; 2012. p. 129–48.

35. Pereira F, Barbachano A, Singh PK, et al. Vitamin D has wide regulatory effects on histone demethylase genes. Cell Cycle 2012;11(6):1081–9.

36. Malireddy S, Kotha SR, Secor JD, et al. Phytochemical antioxidants modulate mammalian cellular epigenome: implications in health and disease. Antioxid Redox Signal 2012;17(2):327–39.

37. Monfort A, Wutz A. Breathing-in epigenetic change with vitamin C. EMBO Rep 2013;14(4):337–46.

38. Hoile SP, Irvine NA, Kelsall CJ, et al. Maternal fat intake in rats alters 20:4n-6 and 22:6n-3 status and the epigenetic regulation of Fads2 in offspring liver. J Nutr Biochem 2013;24(7):1213–20.
39. Remely M, Aumueller E, Merold C, et al. Effects of short chain fatty acid producing bacteria on epigenetic regulation of FFAR3 in type 2 diabetes and obesity. Gene 2014;537(1):85–92.
40. Renz H, Brandtzaeg P, Hornef M. The impact of perinatal immune development on mucosal homeostasis and chronic inflammation. Nat Rev Immunol 2012;12(1):9–23.
41. Anderson OS, Nahar MS, Faulk C, et al. Epigenetic responses following maternal dietary exposure to physiologically relevant levels of bisphenol A. Environ Mol Mutagen 2012;53(5):334–42.
42. Manikkam M, Tracey R, Guerrero-Bosagna C, et al. Plastics derived endocrine disruptors (BPA, DEHP and DBP) induce epigenetic transgenerational inheritance of obesity, reproductive disease and sperm epimutations. PloS One 2013;8(1):e55387.
43. Czeizel AE, Dudas I. Prevention of the first occurrence of neural-tube defects by periconceptional vitamin supplementation. N Engl J Med 1992;327(26):1832–5.
44. Group MVSR. Prevention of neural tube defects: results of the Medical Research Council Vitamin Study. Lancet 1991;338(8760):131–7.
45. Hollingsworth JW, Maruoka S, Boon K, et al. In utero supplementation with methyl donors enhances allergic airway disease in mice. J Clin Invest 2008; 118(10):3462–9.
46. Whitrow MJ, Moore VM, Rumbold AR, et al. Effect of supplemental folic acid in pregnancy on childhood asthma: a prospective birth cohort study. Am J Epidemiol 2009;170(12):1486–93.
47. Dunstan JA, West C, McCarthy S, et al. The relationship between maternal folate status in pregnancy, cord blood folate levels, and allergic outcomes in early childhood. Allergy 2012;67(1):50–7.
48. Crider KS, Cordero AM, Qi YP, et al. Prenatal folic acid and risk of asthma in children: a systematic review and meta-analysis. Am J Clin Nutr 2013;98(5):1272–81.
49. Cho CE, Sanchez-Hernandez D, Reza-Lopez SA, et al. High folate gestational and post-weaning diets alter hypothalamic feeding pathways by DNA methylation in Wistar rat offspring. Epigenetics 2013;8(7):710–9.
50. Utsugi M, Dobashi K, Ishizuka T, et al. c-Jun N-terminal kinase negatively regulates lipopolysaccharide-induced IL-12 production in human macrophages: role of mitogen-activated protein kinase in glutathione redox regulation of IL-12 production. J Immunol 2003;171(2):628–35.
51. Devereux G, Turner SW, Craig LC, et al. Low maternal vitamin E intake during pregnancy is associated with asthma in 5-year-old children. Am J Respir Crit Care Med 2006;174(5):499–507.
52. Martindale S, McNeill G, Devereux G, et al. Antioxidant intake in pregnancy in relation to wheeze and eczema in the first two years of life. Am J Respir Crit Care Med 2005;171(2):121–8.
53. Forastiere F, Pistelli R, Sestini P, et al. Consumption of fresh fruit rich in vitamin C and wheezing symptoms in children. SIDRIA Collaborative Group, Italy (Italian Studies on Respiratory Disorders in Children and the Environment). Thorax 2000;55(4):283–8.
54. Okoko BJ, Burney PG, Newson RB, et al. Childhood asthma and fruit consumption. Eur Respir J 2007;29(6):1161–8.
55. Murr C, Schroecksnadel K, Winkler C, et al. Antioxidants may increase the probability of developing allergic diseases and asthma. Med Hypotheses 2005; 64(5):973–7.

56. Barden AE, Mori TA, Dunstan JA, et al. Fish oil supplementation in pregnancy lowers F2-isoprostanes in neonates at high risk of atopy. Free Radic Res 2004;38(3):233–9.

57. Dunstan JA, Mori TA, Barden A, et al. Fish oil supplementation in pregnancy modifies neonatal allergen-specific immune responses and clinical outcomes in infants at high risk of atopy: a randomized, controlled trial. J Allergy Clin Immunol 2003;112(6):1178–84.

58. Prescott SL, Barden AE, Mori TA, et al. Maternal fish oil supplementation in pregnancy modifies neonatal leukotriene production by cord-blood-derived neutrophils. Clin Sci 2007;113(10):409–16.

59. Furuhjelm C, Warstedt K, Larsson J, et al. Fish oil supplementation in pregnancy and lactation may decrease the risk of infant allergy. Acta Paediatr 2009;98(9):1461–7.

60. Olsen SF, Osterdal ML, Salvig JD, et al. Fish oil intake compared with olive oil intake in late pregnancy and asthma in the offspring: 16 y of registry-based follow-up from a randomized controlled trial. Am J Clin Nutr 2008;88(1):167–75.

61. Palmer DJ, Sullivan T, Gold MS, et al. Effect of n-3 long chain polyunsaturated fatty acid supplementation in pregnancy on infants' allergies in first year of life: randomised controlled trial. BMJ 2012;344:e184.

62. Innis SM. Metabolic programming of long-term outcomes due to fatty acid nutrition in early life. Matern Child Nutr 2011;7(Suppl 2):112–23.

63. Forsyth JS, Willatts P, Agostoni C, et al. Long chain polyunsaturated fatty acid supplementation in infant formula and blood pressure in later childhood: follow up of a randomised controlled trial. BMJ 2003;326(7396):953.

64. Skilton MR, Ayer JG, Harmer JA, et al. Impaired fetal growth and arterial wall thickening: a randomized trial of omega-3 supplementation. Pediatrics 2012;129(3):e698–703.

65. Niculescu MD, Lupu DS, Craciunescu CN. Perinatal manipulation of alpha-linolenic acid intake induces epigenetic changes in maternal and offspring livers. FASEB J 2013;27(1):350–8.

66. Hossein-nezhad A, Holick MF. Optimize dietary intake of vitamin D: an epigenetic perspective. Curr Opin Clin Nutr Metab Care 2012;15(6):567–79.

67. Cordain L, Eaton SB, Sebastian A, et al. Origins and evolution of the Western diet: health implications for the 21st century. Am J Clin Nutr 2005;81(2):341–54.

68. Kuhnlein HV, Receveur O. Dietary change and traditional food systems of indigenous peoples. Annu Rev Nutr 1996;16:417–42.

69. Cani PD, Amar J, Iglesias MA, et al. Metabolic endotoxemia initiates obesity and insulin resistance. Diabetes 2007;56(7):1761–72.

70. Shi L, Li M, Miyazawa K, et al. Effects of heat-inactivated *Lactobacillus gasseri* TMC0356 on metabolic characteristics and immunity of rats with the metabolic syndrome. Br J Nutr 2013;109(2):263–72.

71. Tsukumo DM, Carvalho-Filho MA, Carvalheira JB, et al. Loss-of-function mutation in Toll-like receptor 4 prevents diet-induced obesity and insulin resistance. Diabetes 2007;56(8):1986–98.

72. Renz H. Development and regulation of immune responses in pre- and postnatal life. Clin Biochem 2011;44(7):495.

73. Sudo N, Sawamura S, Tanaka K, et al. The requirement of intestinal bacterial flora for the development of an IgE production system fully susceptible to oral tolerance induction. J Immunol 1997;159(4):1739–45.

74. Turnbaugh PJ, Ley RE, Mahowald MA, et al. An obesity-associated gut microbiome with increased capacity for energy harvest. Nature 2006;444(7122):1027–31.

75. van Hoffen E, Ruiter B, Faber J, et al. A specific mixture of short-chain galacto-ol-igosaccharides and long-chain fructo-oligosaccharides induces a beneficial immunoglobulin profile in infants at high risk for allergy. Allergy 2009;64(3):484–7.

76. Cani PD, Possemiers S, Van de Wiele T, et al. Changes in gut microbiota control inflammation in obese mice through a mechanism involving GLP-2-driven improvement of gut permeability. Gut 2009;58(8):1091–103.

77. Maslowski KM, Vieira AT, Ng A, et al. Regulation of inflammatory responses by gut microbiota and chemoattractant receptor GPR43. Nature 2009;461(7268):1282–6.

78. Maslowski KM, Mackay CR. Diet, gut microbiota and immune responses. Nat Immunol 2011;12(1):5–9.

79. Bottcher MF, Bjorksten B, Gustafson S, et al. Endotoxin levels in Estonian and Swedish house dust and atopy in infancy. Clin Exp Allergy 2003;33(3):295–300.

80. Sjogren YM, Jenmalm MC, Bottcher MF, et al. Altered early infant gut microbiota in children developing allergy up to 5 years of age. Clin Exp Allergy 2009;39(4):518–26.

81. Jenmalm MC, Duchen K. Timing of allergy-preventive and immunomodulatory dietary interventions - are prenatal, perinatal or postnatal strategies optimal? Clin Exp Allergy 2013;43(3):273–8.

82. Prescott SL, Holt PG. Abnormalities in cord blood mononuclear cytokine pro-duction as a predictor of later atopic disease in childhood. Clin Exp Allergy 1998;28(11):1313–6.

83. Tulic MK, Hodder M, Forsberg A, et al. Differences in innate immune function between allergic and nonallergic children: new insights into immune ontogeny. J Allergy Clin Immunol 2011;127(2):470–8.e1.

84. Blumer N, Sel S, Virna S, et al. Perinatal maternal application of *Lactobacillus rhamnosus* GG suppresses allergic airway inflammation in mouse offspring. Clin Exp Allergy 2007;37(3):348–57.

85. Conrad ML, Ferstl R, Teich R, et al. Maternal TLR signaling is required for pre-natal asthma protection by the nonpathogenic microbe *Acinetobacter lwoffii* F78. J Exp Med 2009;206(13):2869–77.

86. Brand S, Teich R, Dicke T, et al. Epigenetic regulation in murine offspring as a novel mechanism for transmaternal asthma protection induced by microbes. J Allergy Clin Immunol 2011;128(3):618–25.e1–7.

87. Rautava S, Collado MC, Salminen S, et al. Probiotics modulate host-microbe interaction in the placenta and fetal gut: a randomized, double-blind, pla-cebo-controlled trial. Neonatology 2012;102(3):178–84.

88. Maurer AD, Reimer RA. Maternal consumption of high-prebiotic fibre or -protein diets during pregnancy and lactation differentially influences satiety hormones and expression of genes involved in glucose and lipid metabolism in offspring in rats. Br J Nutr 2011;105(3):329–38.

89. Fujiwara R, Takemura N, Watanabe J, et al. Maternal consumption of fructo-oligosaccharide diminishes the severity of skin inflammation in offspring of NC/Nga mice. Br J Nutr 2010;103(4):530–8.

90. Shadid R, Haarman M, Knol J, et al. Effects of galactooligosaccharide and long-chain fructooligosaccharide supplementation during pregnancy on maternal and neonatal microbiota and immunity–a randomized, double-blind, placebo-controlled study. Am J Clin Nutr 2007;86(5):1426–37.

91. Gotsis E, Anagnostis P, Mariolis A, et al. Health benefits of the Mediterranean Diet: an update of research over the last 5 years. Angiology 2014, April 27. [Epub ahead of print].

92. Trichopoulou A. Mediterranean diet: the past and the present. Nutrition, metabolism, and cardiovascular diseases. Nutr Metab Cardiovasc Dis 2001;11(4 Suppl):1–4.

Obesity and Asthma
The Role of Environmental Pollutants

Sneha Limaye, MBBS, PDCR*, Sundeep Salvi, MD, DNB, PhD(UK)

KEYWORDS

- Obesity • Air pollution • Endocrine disruptors • Obesogens

KEY POINTS

- Air pollution is a risk factor for obesity.
- Obese individuals are more vulnerable to the harmful effects of air pollutants.
- Obesogens and endocrine-disrupting chemicals is an area for intense research.

Obesity has reached epidemic proportions in both developed as well as developing countries, and high body mass index (BMI) is now recognized as one of the most important determinants of global disease burden.[1,2] It has overtaken tobacco smoking as the most costly and detrimental preventive cause of terminal diseases in the United States.[3] Increases in body weight have also been documented in domesticated, feral, and laboratory animals and urban rats in industrialized countries.[4] In the past, the increase in obesity prevalence has been attributed to excess caloric intake, diet composition, reduction in physical activity, and genetic susceptibility. However, the near doubling in the prevalence of obesity and overweight over the last 3 decades cannot be explained by these traditional factors alone and it has been suggested that additional environmental factors may have contributed to this sudden epidemic.

In 2002, Paula Baillie-Hamilton[5] presented a provocative hypothesis in which she argued that the increase in the prevalence of obesity/overweight in the United States was caused by exposure to environmental toxins. Using evidence from earlier toxicologic studies published in the 1970s, which showed that low-dose chemical exposures were associated with weight gain in experimental animals, she suggested that chemicals present in the air, food, and water altered metabolic processes in the body and led to weight gain. Earlier, in 1991, a multidisciplinary meeting held at the Wingspread Conference Centre in Wisconsin, concerning the magnitude of the problem of endocrine disruptors in the environment, concluded that a large number of human-made chemicals that have been released into the environment, as well as a few natural ones, had the potential to disrupt the endocrine systems of animals, including

Chest Research Foundation, Marigold Premises, Survey No 15, Vadgaonsheri, Kalyaninagar, Pune 411 014, India
* Corresponding author.
E-mail address: snehalimaye@crfindia.com

Immunol Allergy Clin N Am 34 (2014) 839–855
http://dx.doi.org/10.1016/j.iac.2014.07.005
0889-8561/14/$ – see front matter © 2014 Elsevier Inc. All rights reserved.
immunology.theclinics.com

humans. The term endocrine-disrupting chemical (EDC) was coined at this conference, and largely referred to a group of chemicals that had the ability to interfere with the synthesis, secretion, transport, binding action, or elimination of natural hormones in the body and were therefore responsible for disrupting development, behavior, fertility, and cell metabolism.

The World Health Organization (WHO) and the United Nations Environment Program (UNEP) developed a report entitled *Global Assessment of the State of the Science of Endocrine Disruptors* in 2002,[6] which was updated in 2013.[7] This monogram titled *State of the Science of Endocrine Disrupting Chemicals* provides an excellent overview of the current global status of scientific knowledge about EDCs.

In 2006, Grun and Blumberg[8] described the environmental obesogen hypothesis, which postulated a causal link between obesogens (xenobiotic chemicals that can disrupt the normal development and homeostatic controls over adipogenesis and energy balance) in the environment and the obesity epidemic. They had earlier discovered that tin-based compounds known as organotins predisposed laboratory mice to gain weight through an altered endocrine system even when they ate normal food, and suggested that inappropriate activation by organotins causes adipocyte differentiation and a predisposition to obesity.

So far, around 800 EDCs have been described or suspected. However, only a small fraction of these have been studied so far. The known and suspected obesogens include benzo[a]pyrene; particulate matter less than 2.5 μm in mean aerodynamic diameter ($PM_{2.5}$); lead; organic pesticides such as chlorpyrifos, diazinon, and parathion; and industrial chemicals such as bisphenol, organotins, perfluorooctanoic acid (PFOA), phthalates, polybrominated diphenyl ethers (PBDEs), and polychlorinated biphenyl ethers (PCBs) (**Fig. 1**).[9]

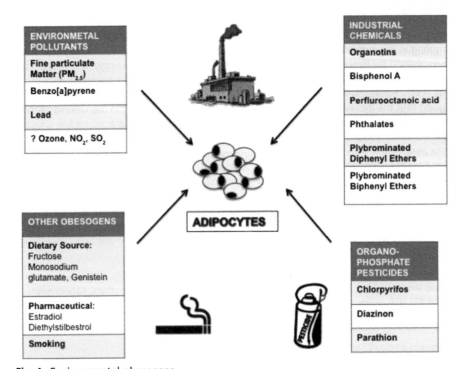

Fig. 1. Environmental obesogens.

Air pollution is now recognized as a risk factor for obesity and at the same time obese individuals are more vulnerable to the harmful effects of air pollution, creating a vicious cycle that may be driving the global obesity epidemic (**Fig. 2**). Early life exposures to environmental chemicals is beginning to be examined as a contributing cause for the obesity epidemic because of the potential critical role of prenatal and perinatal metabolic programming in later risk of obesity.[10] Over the last 5 to 10 years there have been new data for both the epidemiologic evidence linking the effects of environmental chemicals on obesity as well as mechanistic studies designed to elucidate the mechanisms by which these chemicals promote the development of obesity. Many of these, such as tobacco smoke exposure and ambient air pollution, are well-known risks for asthma and this article focuses on how these may also lead to obesity.

AIR POLLUTION AS A RISK FACTOR FOR OBESITY

Epidemiologic Studies

Maternal tobacco smoking and childhood obesity

At least 2 large prospective studies have examined the association between maternal smoking and the risk of obesity in children. In one, 34,866 children born in the United States during 1959 to 1965 were followed more than a period of 8 years and those whose mothers smoked during pregnancy had an increased risk of being overweight by the age of 8 years.[11] In a British birth cohort study that included more than 5800 boys and girls, children of mothers who smoked during pregnancy were lighter at birth than children of nonsmokers, but from adolescence (age 11 years for girls, and 16 years for boys) they had an increased risk of being in the highest deciles of BMI. The odds ratios for obesity associated with maternal smoking increased with age, suggesting strengthening of the relationship over time. At age 33 years the odds ratio was 1.56 (95% confidence interval [CI], 1.22–2.00) for men and 1.41 (95% CI, 1.12–1.79) for women. This increased risk was robust to adjustment for factors in early life, childhood, and adulthood.[12]

An environmental study in 1983 reported that higher plasma benzo[a]pyrene concentrations were associated with a higher BMI in human subjects living in New York.[13] Since then, several cross-sectional studies have shown that childhood obesity is associated with maternal smoking during pregnancy.[14] In a population-based cohort of 3253 children from Brisbane, Australia, the prevalence of overweight and obesity among adolescents was greater among those whose mothers smoked during pregnancy.[15]

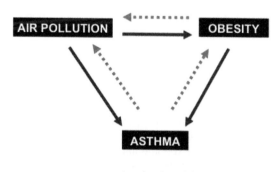

Fig. 2. Vicious cycle of obesity epidemic.

Ambient air pollution and obesity

A longitudinal study in 3318 children from Southern California reported a significant positive association between proximity and density of truck traffic and the BMI of children over an 8-year follow-up period.[16] As the distance of residence increased, the odds of children becoming overweight reduced. More recently, long-term exposure to vehicular traffic, as estimated by proximity of residence to highways, was shown to be positively associated with increased insulin resistance in children.[17] Rajagopalan and Brook[18] reviewed 6 published studies from Canada, Germany, the United States, Denmark, Iran, and Taiwan that showed an association between particulate matter or traffic-related air pollutants and diabetes. A 10-μg/m^3 increase in PM$_{2.5}$ was reported to be associated with a 1% increase in the prevalence of diabetes,[19] or exposures to nitrogen dioxide and PM$_{10}$ were associated with a 4% to 42% increased risk of diabetes.[20,21] In Taiwan, increases in annual PM$_{2.5}$ levels by 35 μg/m^3 were related to increases in glucose and hemoglobin A1c levels.[22]

Given the billions of people continuously exposed and the rapid industrial/urban growth among developing nations, even a modest causal association would be of major public health importance.

Other air pollutants and obesity

La Merrill and Birnbaum[10] reviewed existing prospective and cross-sectional studies that examined the association between maternal exposures to various EDCs, including organochlorine pesticides (dichlorodiphenyltrichloroethane [DDT], dichloro-diphenyldichloroethylene [DDE], and hexachlorobenzene), dioxinlike compounds (toxic equivalent quantity of polychlorinated dibenzodioxin, polychlorinated dibenzo-furan, PCB118, dioxinlike PCBs), and nondioxinlike PCBs. Four of the 5 prospective studies and 5 of the 6 cross-sectional studies reported that maternal exposures to DDT and DDE during pregnancy were associated with increased obesity in children. In a longitudinal birth cohort study in Salinas, California, Warner and colleagues[23] reported a significant association between prenatal exposure to DDT and DDE and several measures of obesity at 9 years of age in boys but not in girls. A 10-fold increase in prenatal DDT exposure was associated with 2.5-fold increased odds of becoming overweight or obese. **Fig. 3** shows the different EDCs and their sources.[24]

Mechanistic Studies on How Air Pollution Causes Obesity

The molecular mechanisms by which air pollution cause obesity remain poorly understood. Exposure to air pollutants occurs even before people are born. Laboratory tests commissioned by the Environmental Working Group (EWG) in the United States detected bisphenol A (BPA), a known EDC, for the first time in 9 out of 10 umbilical cord blood samples of US babies born between December 2007 and June 2008 in Michigan, Florida, Massachusetts, California, and Wisconsin.[25] Additional tests conducted by 5 laboratories in the United States, Canada, and Europe found up to 232 toxic chemicals in the 10 cord blood samples. Besides BPA, substances detected for the first time in umbilical cord blood included a toxic flame retardant chemical tetrabromobisphenol A, which permeates computer circuit boards; synthetic fragrances used in common cosmetics and detergents; and perfluorobutanoic acid, a member of the notorious Teflon chemical family used to make nonstick and grease-resistant, stain-resistant, and water-resistant coatings for cookware, textiles, food packaging, and other consumer products. Experimental as well as human exposure studies indicate that the growing fetus is more sensitive than adults to diverse environmental toxicants, including lead, mercury, environmental tobacco smoke, polyaromatic hydrocarbons (PAHs), and residential pesticides such as diazinon and

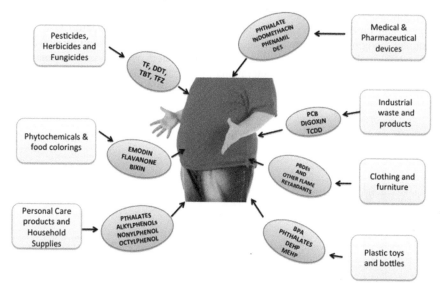

Fig. 3. EDCs and their sources. BPA, bisphenol A; DEHP, di-2-ethylhexyl phthalate; DES, diethylstilbestrol; MEHP, monoethylhexyl phthalate; TBT, tributyltin; TF, tolylfluanid; TFZ, triflumizole.

chlorpyrifospesticides.[26–29] Exposure to many of these pollutants during fetal growth has been shown to produce metabolic reprogramming in the fetus that leads to subsequent risk of obesity.[30,31]

The growing fetus does not have the protective mechanisms of an adult, such as DNA repair mechanisms, a fully competent immune system, detoxifying enzymes, and liver metabolism. Moreover, the developing fetus has a greater metabolic rate compared with an adult. These factors make the growing fetus more sensitive to chemical toxicity. Exposures to certain environmental chemicals during critical periods of differentiation can cause adverse effects, some of which may not be apparent until later in life.[32]

Tobacco smoke and lipids

One study reported that in utero exposure to tobacco smoke was associated with greater levels of serum cholesterol during adulthood.[33,34] More recently, the Norwegian Mother and Child Cohort Study reported that exposure to tobacco smoke in utero was associated with a 2.5-fold greater risk of having increased triglycerides (CI, 1.3–5.1) and a 2.3-fold risk of having low high-density lipoprotein levels (CI, 1.1–5.0) when examined 18 to 44 years later.[35]

Epigenetic changes Environmental exposures have been shown to be associated with epigenetic changes. Arsenic, one of the heavy metals found in cigarette smoke, has been shown to be associated with global DNA hypomethylation, in both in vitro studies[36] and animal experiments.[37] Two retrospective studies have shown an association between in utero exposure to tobacco smoke and global DNA hypomethylation.[38,39]

More recently, Guerrero-Preston and colleagues[40] studied global DNA methylation in newborns and its association with exposure to maternal smoking. They also measured association between levels of DNA methylation and persistent perfluoroalkyl

compounds (PFCs) in cord serum. They reported increase in global DNA hypomethylation in the umbilical cord serum, which was significantly associated in a dose-
response fashion to in utero exposure to tobacco smoke. They also reported that
DNA global methylation in cord serum was associated with prenatal exposure to
PFCs, especially PFOA (**Fig. 4**). Alterations in the global DNA methylation patterns

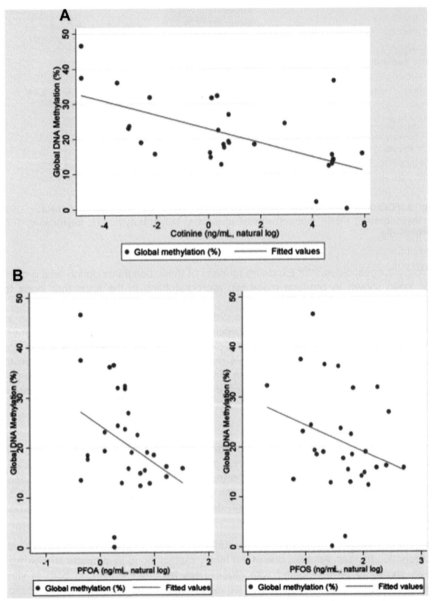

Fig. 4. (A) Linear relationship between cord blood serum and the global DNA methylation
index. (B) Linear relationship between the natural log of PFOA (perfluorooctanoate). (*From*
Guerrero-Preston R, Goldman LR, Brebi-Mieville P, et al. Global DNA hypomethylation is
associated with in utero exposure to cotinine and perfluorinated alkyl compounds. Epigenetics 2010;5:543. http://dx.doi.org/10.4161/epi.5.6.12378; with permission.)

have been associated with various human diseases that could contribute to obesity, such as cancer,[41] hypertension,[42] cardiovascular disease,[43] autoimmune disease,[44] and more recently with insulin resistance.[45]

Polyaromatic Hydrocarbons and Estrogenic Activity

Polyaromatic hydrocarbons are air pollutants commonly generated from motor vehicular exhausts, especially from diesel vehicles, and can easily cross the placental barrier after being inhaled by the pregnant mother. Hydroxy-PAHs are structurally similar to estrogen and have been shown to have estrogenic activity in breast adenoma cell lines.[46] PAHs have been shown to alter estrogen signaling through crosstalk between the estrogen receptor and the aryl hydrocarbon receptor, for which PAHs are ligands.[47] Prenatal and early life exposure to environmental estrogens has been shown to cause obesity later in life.[48] Children born to African American and Hispanic mothers living in the Bronx or northern Manhattan in New York who were followed up to the age of 7 years had a strong association between obesity and indoor or personal PAH levels of their mothers when they were in the womb, indicating that prenatal exposure to PAHs is associated with obesity in childhood.[49] In utero exposure to PAH was associated with a 79% greater risk of obesity at the age of 5 years and 226% at the age of 7 years even after correcting for potential confounding factors such as socioeconomic status (**Fig. 5**).

Inflammation and Adipose Tissue

One of the mechanisms by which air pollution has been shown to induce obesity is via a systemic inflammatory pathway that targets adipocytes. Exposure to $PM_{2.5}$ pollutants has been shown to cause visceral adipose tissue inflammation and oxidative stress, along with alterations in the levels of circulating adipokines, including adiponectin and leptin,[50] suggesting that the adipose tissue may be a critical target for metabolic disruption by the EDCs. The adipose tissue is a dynamic organ that is

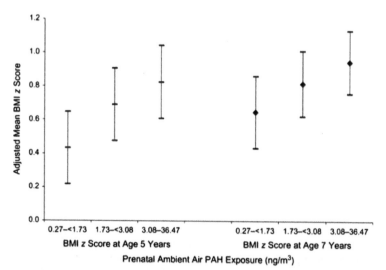

Fig. 5. Covariate-adjusted mean BMI according to tertile of prenatal ambient air PAH exposure for children. (*Adapted from* Rundle A, Hoepner L, Hassoun A, et al. Association of childhood obesity with maternal exposure to ambient air polycyclic aromatic hydrocarbons during pregnancy. Am J Epidemiol 2012;175:1169; with permission.)

centrally involved in the integrative network that maintains global energy homeostasis. Many classes of EDCs have been shown to be highly lipophilic and therefore to accumulate in the lipid droplets of mature adipocytes, resulting in high local concentration in the fat pad.[51] Bioaccumulation of EDCs in the adipose tissue may result in sustained local exposure and signaling that not only may release proinflammatory signals but may cause further adipocyte proliferation and differentiation. Furthermore, the accumulated EDCs in the adipose tissue can be released back into the systemic circulation, thereby influencing the function of other metabolic tissues.

Rats exposed to oraganophosphorus insecticides, such as chlorpyrifos, have been shown to develop increased adipose tissue at doses that do not produce symptoms of acute cholinesterase inhibition.[52] In neonatal rats, organophosphate exposure during a critical developmental window has been shown to alter the trajectory of hepatic adenylyl cyclase/cyclic adenosine monophosphate signaling, culminating in hyperresponsiveness to gluconeogenic stimuli. These animals consequently developed metabolic dysfunction resembling prediabetes. When the organophosphate-exposed animals consumed a high-fat diet in adulthood, metabolic defects were exacerbated and animals gained excess weight compared with unexposed rats on the same diet.[53]

Liu and colleagues[54] recently reported that mice exposed to $PM_{2.5}$ pollutants produced insulin resistance by regulating visceral adipose tissue inflammation, hepatic lipid metabolism, and glucose use in skeletal muscle via both CCR2-dependent and CCR2-independent pathways, providing potential metabolic abnormalities underlying insulin resistance. The same group reported that a 10-month chronic exposure to $PM_{2.5}$ in mice induced macrophage infiltration and unfolded protein response in the white adipose tissue,[55] mediated early alterations in insulin resistance, and caused visceral inflammation and structural and functional alterations in the brown adipose tissue.[56,57] Along with the endoplasmic reticular stress response, expression of the genes involved in lipogenesis, lipolysis, adipocyte differentiation, and lipid droplet formation increased in the white adipose tissue of the mice exposed to $PM_{2.5}$.[55] It has been suggested that inflammation, oxidative stress and endoplasmic reticular stress response are likely integrated in the liver and adipose tissue, from where they may form a stress loop that contributes to alteration in lipid and energy metabolism following exposure to EDCs such as $PM_{2.5}$ pollutants.[58]

One of the EDCs, PCB77 (3,3′,4,4′-tetrachlorobiphenyl), has been shown to increase adipocyte differentiation, promote expression of proinflammatory cytokines, and augment the expression of peroxisome proliferator–activated receptor gamma, a key promoter in regulating cell energy homeostasis.[59] Many of these chemicals have been shown to be capable of accumulating in the human body throughout the lifespan.[60,61]

Effects on Endocrine and Autonomic Nervous System

Environmental toxins such as heavy metals, solvents, polychlorinated biphenols, organophosphates, phthalates, and bisphenol A have been shown to induce obesity via alterations in weight-controlling hormones, alterations in sensitivity to neurotransmitters, or alterations in the activity of the sympathetic nervous system. EDCs have been shown to activate the hypothalamo-pituitary-adrenal (HPA) axis that could lead to obesity, although the mechanism is not known.[62] Inhaled pollutants from the lungs can enter the systemic circulation and get deposited in other body organs.[63] Some studies have suggested that inhaled pollutants may reach the brain and stimulate local production of prostaglandins in the pituitary.[64,65]

Animal studies have shown that prenatal exposure to nicotine causes weight gain by disrupting the cholinergic and catecholaminergic systems.[66] Modulation of the sympathetic nervous system by the EDCs has been proposed to cause weight gain. For example, benzo[a]pyrenes have been shown to have properties simulating β-blockers. Chronic exposure of mice to benzo[a]pyrene for 15 days has been shown to reduce lipolytic responses to epinephrine and cause a 43% weight gain compared with controls, without any detectable changes in food intake. Similar inhibition of beta-adrenergic receptors has been reported in human isolated adipocytes.[67] The same investigators reported that mice exposed to benzo[a]pyrene for 2 weeks showed a significant decrease in the expression of β1-adrenergic and β2-adrenergic receptors, lipoprotein lipase, and diacylglycerol acyltransferase in adipose tissue.

OBESITY INCREASES VULNERABILITY TO THE HARMFUL EFFECTS OF AIR POLLUTION

Obesity is a recognized risk factor for cardiovascular diseases.[68] It causes various pathophysiologic changes that make obese individuals more vulnerable to developing cardiovascular comorbid conditions. The underlying morbid state present in obesity is further amplified after exposure to air pollutants, making obese individuals more vulnerable to the harmful effects of air pollution than lean individuals. This greater vulnerability is highlighted by 3 large observational prospective cohort studies. Miller and colleagues[69] studied 65,893 postmenopausal women without previous cardiovascular diseases in 36 US metropolitan areas over a mean follow-up period of 6 years, and reported that women with the highest BMI had an 84% increased risk of cardiovascular events compared with those with the lowest BMI for the same level of exposure to ambient air pollutants. Puett and colleagues[70] prospectively followed up 66,250 nurses in the United States for a period of 10 years and studied the relationships between ambient $PM_{2.5}$ levels and incident coronary heart disease (CHD), fatal CHD, and nonfatal myocardial infarction (MI). Increased levels of ambient $PM_{2.5}$ were strongly associated with increased risk of fatal CHD and nonfatal MI, and the magnitude of this association was 3-fold greater among obese subjects. Weichenthal and colleagues[71] similarly followed up 5931 US farmers over a period of 14 years and reported that farmers in the highest BMI category had a greater than 2-fold increased risk of cardiovascular mortality than lean individuals for the same levels of exposure to $PM_{2.5}$.

Obese individuals are more vulnerable to developing respiratory disorders following exposure to air pollutants than lean individuals, which has recently been highlighted by 2 longitudinal cohort studies. The Veterans Administration Normative Aging Study was a 10-year longitudinal cohort study among 904 elderly men that examined the interactions between obesity and ambient levels of ozone every 3 years during the preceding 48 hours of lung function.[72] An increase in ambient ozone levels of 15 ppb was associated with a greater decline in lung function as measured by spirometry, an effect that was more pronounced among obese individuals, indicating that obesity modified the acute effects of ozone air pollution on lung function in the elderly. In another prospective cohort study, 148 children aged 5 to 17 years with persistent asthma were followed for 1 year during which associations between indoor $PM_{2.5}$ and nitrogen dioxide (NO_2) levels and respiratory symptoms were examined every 3 months.[73] Overweight children were more susceptible to the pulmonary effects of indoor $PM_{2.5}$ and NO_2, and it was suggested that the combination of a high prevalence of overweight status and high indoor pollutant exposure in urban children with asthma could explain some of the disproportionate asthma morbidity seen in this population.

Several cross-sectional studies have also examined the vulnerability of obese individuals to respiratory disorders following exposure to air pollutants. The Seven North Eastern Cities (SNEC) was a cross-sectional study in China that investigated the effects of ambient air pollution on children[74] and reported that ambient levels of air pollutants were associated with adverse respiratory symptoms among children, and that obese and overweight children had a more pronounced effect. Obese asthmatic as well as nonasthmatic human subjects exposed to controlled 0.42-ppm ozone for 1.5 hours were shown to produce greater decrements in lung function than lean individuals.[75] A recent study in asthmatic individuals aged 65 years and older also reported that the mean daily concentration of elemental carbon was associated with poorer asthma control among obese, but not among nonobese, asthmatics, suggesting that obesity can modify the effects of air pollutants on asthma exacerbations.[76] More recently, Jung and colleagues[77] measured indoor levels of polyaromatic hydrocarbons in the homes of children aged 5 to 6 years and studied their association with childhood asthma. Higher concentrations of PAHs were associated with asthma among obese children, but not among nonobese children.

Although epidemiologic studies help establish associations, they do not establish causality. Causal inference can be further strengthened by the presence of underlying biological mechanisms. Why obese individuals are more vulnerable to the harmful effects of air pollutants has been a subject of intense research and several novel potential mechanisms have recently been described.

Obesity increases the stiffening of the respiratory system as well as the mechanical work needed for breathing,[78,79] which contributes to smaller lung volumes than are found in normal-weight individuals.[80] In addition, owing to changes in the structure of the lungs, obese individuals have a reduced functional residual capacity.[81] Moreover, obese individuals breathe with smaller tidal volumes than individuals of normal weight, which leads to a reduction in lung tissue stretching that could potentially affect sensitivity to ambient air pollution.[74] Overall, obesity has been shown to affect respiratory resistance, lung volumes, spirometric measures, bronchial hyperreactivity, upper airway mechanical function, neuromuscular strength, and the lung diffusing capacity.[78]

An earlier study by Shore and colleagues[82] reported that obese mice inhaled greater doses of the air pollutant ozone into the lungs than normal-weight mice because of their higher breathing frequency. This finding was accompanied by greater airway hyperresponsiveness and greater cellular inflammation in the airways of obese mice. A subsequent inhalation study in healthy children aged 6 to 13 years reported that children with the highest BMI had a 2.8-times greater deposition of fine particles into the lungs than the leanest children for the same amount of air pollution exposure (Kim Lu et al). An earlier study showed similar observations in obese adults.[83] The sedentary lifestyles of obese individuals means that they spend greater amounts of their time indoors, where substantial semivolatile PAH sources are present, thereby increasing their exposure to various indoor air pollutants.

Obesity is a proinflammatory state. Adipose tissue is known to express several proinflammatory molecules, including tumor necrosis factor alpha (TNFα), in a pattern that could be analogous to the immune function of T lymphocytes and macrophages. When exposed to air pollutants the inflammatory response may be further amplified, thereby increasing the vulnerability of obese subjects to the harmful respiratory effects. Inhaled particulate pollutants phagocytosed by the alveolar macrophages in the airways secrete TNFα in a dose-dependent manner. These cells also produce interleukin (IL)-6, IL-1β, and granulocyte-macrophage colony-stimulating factor, cytokines that spill into the systemic circulation and can mount a systemic inflammatory response. Obese individuals exposed to air pollutants have been shown to mount a greater increase in the levels of serum C-reactive proteins[84] and circulating soluble vascular adhesion molecule-1[85] (a marker of endothelial dysfunction and inflammation) than lean subjects.

Lungs of obese mice exposed to ozone have been shown to produce a greater increase in IL-6 levels associated with greater neutrophil influx compared with lean mice.[86] Leptin, a member of the IL-6 family of cytokines produced by adipocytes, has been shown to enhance ozone-induced airway hyperresponsiveness and induce neutrophil influx. Increased serum leptin levels have been shown to be associated with greater levels of the chemokine macrophage inflammatory protein-2 following acute ozone exposure, and suggest that the proinflammatory effects of leptin may contribute to increased susceptibility of obese individuals to air pollutants.[87]

Obesity is also associated with increased systemic oxidative stress. Excess glucose has been shown to stimulate the generation of reactive oxygen species (ROS). The superoxide radicals further activate the redox-sensitive proinflammatory transcription factor nuclear factor kappa B, which has the potential to activate the transcription of several proinflammatory genes. Dietary restriction and weight loss have been shown to produce significant reductions in oxidative stress. For example, a 48-hour fast has been shown to produce an almost 50% reduction in ROS generation by leukocytes and a diminution in the expression of Nicotinamide adenine dinucleotide phosphate hydrogen oxidase, the enzyme that converts molecular oxygen to the superoxide radical.[88] Air pollutants, including particulate matter, have been shown to produce oxidative stress.[89] The existing systemic oxidative stress in obese asthmatics may make them more susceptible to the harmful effects of air pollution by further exacerbating systemic oxidative responses in the lungs. **Fig. 6** provides a summary of different mechanisms through which obesity increases the susceptibility of an individual to harmful effects of air pollution. These effects coupled with the existing compromised defense system of the lungs in asthma lead to an exaggerated effect of air pollutants on obese asthmatics.

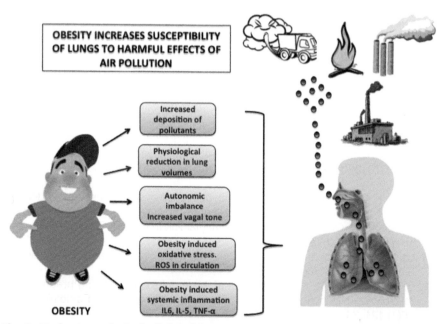

Fig. 6. Mechanisms of obesity-induced increased susceptibility to harmful effects of air pollutants.

SUMMARY

Air pollution is now recognized as a novel risk factor for the development of obesity. Longitudinal as well as cross-sectional studies have established an association between various ambient and indoor air pollutants and obesity or increased BMI. Several xenobiotic chemicals that can disrupt the normal development and homeostatic controls over adipogenesis and energy balance, called obesogens, have been identified, exposures to which have been shown to induce obesity. Several animal exposure studies and laboratory studies have suggested novel underlying mechanisms that drive the development of obesity. In contrast, obese individuals are also more vulnerable to the harmful effects of air pollutants than lean individuals and this drives a vicious cycle promoting more obesity. Several mechanisms have been proposed that increase this vulnerability. Despite the emerging evidence for the role of air pollutants in obesity, this topic is still in its infancy. More knowledge needs to be generated by means of dose-response studies on air pollutants and obesity to conclusively establish the link.

REFERENCES

1. WHO. World Health Organization fact sheet (number 311) for worldwide prevalence of obesity. 2013. Available at: http://www.who.int/mediacentre/factsheets/fs311/en/. Accessed May 12, 2014.
2. Lim S, Vos T, Flaxman AD, et al. A comparative risk assessment of burden of disease and injury attributable to 67 risk factors and risk factor clusters in 21 regions, 1990–2010: A systematic analysis for the Global Burden of Disease Study 2010. Lancet 2012;380:2224–60.
3. Cawley J, Meyerhoefer C. The medical care costs of obesity: an instrumental variables approach. J Health Econ 2012;31(1):219–30.
4. Klimentidis Y, Beasley T, Lin H, et al. Canaries in the coal mine: a cross-species analysis of the plurality of obesity epidemics. Proc Biol Sci 2011;278(1712):1626–32.
5. Baillie-Hamilton PF. Chemical toxins: a hypothesis to explain the global obesity epidemic. J Altern Complement Med 2002;8(2):185–92.
6. Damstra T, Barlow S, Bergman A, et al, editors. World Health Organization and United Nations Environment Programme. Global assessment of the state-of-the-science of endocrine disruptors. WHO; 2002. Available at: www.who.int/ipcs/publications/en/toc.pdf?ua=1.
7. Bergman A, Heindel H, Jobling S, et al, editors. World Health Organization and United Nations Environment Programme. State of the science of endocrine disrupting chemicals – 2012. WHO; 2012. Available at: http://apps.who.int/iris/bitstream/10665/78102/1/WHO_HSE_PHE_IHE_2013.1_eng.pdf?ua=1. Accessed May 15, 2014.
8. Grun F, Blumberg B. Environmental obesogens: organotins and endocrine disruption via nuclear receptor signaling. Endocrinology 2006;147(6):s50–5.
9. Holtcamp W. Obesogens: an environmental link to obesity. Environ Health Perspect 2012;120(2):a62.
10. La Merrill M, Birnbaum L. Childhood obesity and environmental chemicals. Mt Sinai J Med 2011;78(1):22–48.
11. Chen A, Pennell M, Klebanoff M, et al. Maternal smoking during pregnancy in relation to child overweight: follow-up to age 8 years. Int J Epidemiol 2006;35(1):121–30.
12. Power C, Jefferis B. Fetal environment and subsequent obesity: a study of maternal smoking. Int J Epidemiol 2002;31(2):413–9.

13. Hutcheon D, Kantrowitz J, Van Gelder R, et al. Factors affecting plasma benzo[a]pyrene levels in environmental studies. Environ Res 1983;32(1): 104–10.
14. Toschke A, Koletzko B, Slikker W, et al. Childhood obesity is associated with maternal smoking in pregnancy. Eur J Pediatr 2002;161(8):445–8.
15. Al Mamun A, Lawlor D, Alati R, et al. Does maternal smoking during pregnancy have a direct effect on future offspring obesity? Evidence from a prospective birth cohort study. Am J Epidemiol 2006;164(4):317–25.
16. Jerrett M, McConnell R, Chang C, et al. Automobile traffic around the home and attained body mass index: a longitudinal cohort study of children aged 10–18 years. Prev Med 2010;50:S50–8.
17. Thiering E, Cyrys J, Kratzsch J, et al. Long-term exposure to traffic-related air pollution and insulin resistance in children: results from the GINIplus and LISA-plus birth cohorts. Diabetologia 2013;56(8):1696–704.
18. Rajagopalan S, Brook R. Air pollution and type 2 diabetes mechanistic insights. Diabetes 2012;61(12):3037–45.
19. Pearson J, Bachireddy C, Shyamprasad S, et al. Association between fine particulate matter and diabetes prevalence in the US. Diabetes Care 2010;33(10): 2196–201.
20. Brook RD, Jerrett M, Brook JR, et al. The relationship between diabetes mellitus and traffic-related air pollution. J Occup Environ Med 2008;50:32–8.
21. Krämer U, Herder C, Sugiri D, et al. Traffic-related air pollution and incident type 2 diabetes: results from the SALIA cohort study. Environ Health Perspect 2010; 118(9):1273.
22. Chuang K, Yan Y, Chiu S, et al. Long-term air pollution exposure and risk factors for cardiovascular diseases among the elderly in Taiwan. Occup Environ Med 2011;68(1):64–8.
23. Warner M, Wesselink A, Harley K, et al. Prenatal exposure to dichlorodiphenyl-trichloroethane and obesity at 9 years of age in the CHAMACOS Study Cohort. Am J Epidemiol 2014;179(11):1312–22.
24. Regnier S, Sargis R. Adipocytes under assault: environmental disruption of adipose physiology. Biochim Biophys Acta 2014;1842(3):520–33.
25. Buchanan S, Rizzo J, Rolfes A, et al. Toxic chemicals found in minority cord blood. EWG Public Affairs. Available at: http://www.ewg.org/news/news-releases/2009/12/02/toxic-chemicals-found-minority-cord-blood. Accessed May 15, 2014.
26. National Research Council (US), Committee on Pesticides in the Diets of Infants, Children. Pesticides in the diets of infants and children. Washington DC: National Academy Press; 1993.
27. Perera F, Tang D, Rauh V, et al. Relationships among polycyclic aromatic hydrocarbon–DNA adducts, proximity to the World Trade Center, and effects on fetal growth. Environ Health Perspect 2005;113(8):1062.
28. Whyatt R, Perera F. Application of biologic markers to studies of environmental risks in children and the developing fetus. Environ Health Perspect 1995; 103(Suppl 6):105.
29. World Health Organization (Geneva). Principles for evaluating health risks from chemicals during infancy and early childhood: the need for a special approach/ published under the joint sponsorship of the United Nations Environment Programme, the International Labour Organization, the World Health Organization, and on behalf of the Commission of the European Communities. 1986.
30. Bruin J, Gerstein H, Holloway A. Long-term consequences of fetal and neonatal nicotine exposure: a critical review. Toxicol Sci 2010;116(2):364–74.

31. Gluckman P, Hanson M. The developmental origins of the metabolic syndrome. Trends Endocrinol Metab 2004;15(4):183–7.
32. Newbold R, Padilla-Banks E, Jefferson W. Environmental estrogens and obesity. Mol Cell Endocrinol 2009;304(1):84–9.
33. Jaddoe V, de Ridder M, van den Elzen A, et al. Maternal smoking in pregnancy is associated with cholesterol development in the offspring: a 27-years follow-up study. Atherosclerosis 2008;196(1):42–8.
34. Wen X, Triche E, Hogan J, et al. Birth weight and adult hypercholesterolemia: subgroups of small-for-gestational-age based on maternal smoking status during pregnancy. Epidemiology 2010;21(6):786–90.
35. Cupul-Uicab L, Skjaerven R, Haug K, et al. Exposure to tobacco smoke in utero and subsequent plasma lipids, ApoB, and CRP among adult women in the MoBa cohort. Environ Health Perspect 2012;120(11):1532.
36. Jensen T, Novak P, Wnek S, et al. Arsenicals produce stable progressive changes in DNA methylation patterns that are linked to malignant transformation of immortalized urothelial cells. Toxicol Appl Pharmacol 2009;241(2):221–9.
37. Chen H, Li S, Liu J, et al. Chronic inorganic arsenic exposure induces hepatic global and individual gene hypomethylation: implications for arsenic hepatocarcinogenesis. Carcinogenesis 2004;25(9):1779–86.
38. Terry M, Ferris J, Pilsner R, et al. Genomic DNA methylation among women in a multiethnic New York City birth cohort. Cancer Epidemiol Biomarkers Prev 2008; 17(9):2306–10.
39. Breton C, Byun H, Wenten M, et al. Prenatal tobacco smoke exposure affects global and gene-specific DNA methylation. Am J Respir Crit Care Med 2009; 180(5):462.
40. Guerrero-Preston R, Goldman L, Brebi-Mieville P, et al. Global DNA hypomethylation is associated with in utero exposure to cotinine and perfluorinated alkyl compounds. Epigenetics 2010;5(6):539.
41. Chalitchagorn K, Shuangshoti S, Hourpai N, et al. Distinctive pattern of LINE-1 methylation level in normal tissues and the association with carcinogenesis. Oncogene 2004;23:8841–6.
42. Smolarek I, Wyszko E, Barciszewska A, et al. Global DNA methylation changes in blood of patients with essential hypertension. Med Sci Monit 2010;16(3): CR149–55.
43. Kim M, Long T, Arakawa K, et al. DNA methylation as a biomarker for cardiovascular disease risk. PLoS One 2010;5(3):e9692.
44. Liu C, Ou T, Wu C, et al. Global DNA methylation, DNMT1, and MBD2 in patients with systemic lupus erythematosus. Lupus 2011;20(2):131–6.
45. Zhao J, Goldberg J, Bremner JD, et al. Global DNA methylation is associated with insulin resistance a monozygotic twin study. Diabetes 2012;61(2):542–6.
46. Wenger D, Gerecke A, Heeb N, et al. In vitro estrogenicity of ambient particulate matter: contribution of hydroxylated polycyclic aromatic hydrocarbons. J Appl Toxicol 2009;29(3):223–32.
47. Safe S, Wormke M. Inhibitory aryl hydrocarbon receptor-estrogen receptor α cross-talk and mechanisms of action. Chem Res Toxicol 2003;16(7):807–16.
48. Newbold R, Padilla-Banks E, Snyder R, et al. Perinatal exposure to environmental estrogens and the development of obesity. Mol Nutr Food Res 2007; 51(7):912–7.
49. Rundle A, Hoepner L, Hassoun A, et al. Association of childhood obesity with maternal exposure to ambient air polycyclic aromatic hydrocarbons during pregnancy. Am J Epidemiol 2012;175(11):1163–72.

50. Xu Z, Xu X, Zhong M, et al. Ambient particulate air pollution induces oxidative stress and alterations of mitochondria and gene expression in brown and white adipose tissues. Part Fibre Toxicol 2011;8:20.
51. Sargis R, Neel B, Brock C, et al. The novel endocrine disruptor tolylfluanid impairs insulin signaling in primary rodent and human adipocytes through a reduction in insulin receptor substrate-1 levels. Biochim Biophys Acta 2012;1822(6): 952–60.
52. Meggs J, Kori L. Weight gain associated with chronic exposure to chlorpyrifos in rats. J Med Toxicol 2007;3(3):89–93.
53. Slotkin TA. Does early-life exposure to organophosphate insecticides lead to prediabetes and obesity? Reprod Toxicol 2011;31:297–301.
54. Liu C, Xu X, Bai Y, et al. Air pollution-mediated susceptibility to inflammation and insulin resistance: influence of CCR2 pathways in mice. Environ Health Perspect 2014;122(1):17–26.
55. Mendez R, Zheng Z, Fan Z, et al. Exposure to fine airborne particulate matter induces macrophage infiltration, unfolded protein response, and lipid deposition in white adipose tissue. Am J Transl Res 2013;5(2):224.
56. Sun Q, Yue P, Deiuliis J, et al. Ambient air pollution exaggerates adipose inflammation and insulin resistance in a mouse model of diet-induced obesity. Circulation 2009;119(4):538–46.
57. Xu X, Liu C, Xu Z, et al. Long-term exposure to ambient fine particulate pollution induces insulin resistance and mitochondrial alteration in adipose tissue. Toxicol Sci 2011;124(1):88–98.
58. Chen J, Brown T, Russo J. Regulation of energy metabolism pathways by estrogens and estrogenic chemicals and potential implications in obesity associated with increased exposure to endocrine disruptors. Biochim Biophys Acta 2009; 1793(7):1128–43.
59. Arsenescu V, Arsenescu R, King V, et al. Polychlorinated biphenyl-77 induces adipocyte differentiation and proinflammatory adipokines and promotes obesity and atherosclerosis. Environ Health Perspect 2008;116(6):761.
60. Lee A, Hiscock R, Wein P, et al. Gestational diabetes mellitus: clinical predictors and long-term risk of developing type 2 diabetes a retrospective cohort study using survival analysis. Diabetes Care 2007;30(4):878–83.
61. Hue O, Marcotte J, Berrigan F, et al. Plasma concentration of organochlorine compounds is associated with age and not obesity. Chemosphere 2007;67(7): 1463–7.
62. Janesick A, Blumberg B. Obesogens, stem cells and the developmental programming of obesity. Int J Androl 2012;35(3):437–48.
63. Oberdörster G, Sharp Z, Atudorei V, et al. Translocation of inhaled ultrafine particles to the brain. Inhal Toxicol 2004;16(6-7):437–45.
64. Bugajski J, Gadek-Michalska A, Bugajski A. Nitric oxide and prostaglandin systems in the stimulation of hypothalamic-pituitary-adrenal axis by neurotransmitters and neurohormones. J Physiol Pharmacol 2004;55(4):679.
65. Reimsnider S, Wood C. Co-localisation of prostaglandin endoperoxide synthase and immunoreactive adrenocorticotrophic hormone in ovine foetal pituitary. J Endocrinol 2004;180(2):303–10.
66. Levin ED. Animal models of developmental nicotine exposure: possible mechanisms of childhood obesity. Birth Defects Research Part E 2003;68(3):245.
67. Irigaray P, Ogier V, Jacquenet S, et al. Benzo[a]pyrene impairs beta-adrenergic stimulation of adipose tissue lipolysis and causes weight gain in mice. FEBS J 2006;273(7):1362–72.

68. Hubert H, Feinleib M, McNamara P, et al. Obesity as an independent risk factor for cardiovascular disease: a 26-year follow-up of participants in the Framingham Heart Study. Circulation 1983;67(5):968–77.

69. Miller K, Siscovick D, Sheppard L, et al. Long-term exposure to air pollution and incidence of cardiovascular events in women. N Engl J Med 2007;356: 447–58.

70. Puett R, Hart J, Yanosky J, et al. Chronic fine and coarse particulate exposure, mortality, and coronary heart disease in the Nurses' Health Study. Environ Health Perspect 2009;117:1697–701.

71. Weichenthal S, Villeneuve P, Burnett R, et al. Long-term exposure to fine particulate matter: association with non-accidental and cardiovascular mortality in the agricultural health study cohort. Environ Health Perspect 2014. http://dx.doi.org/ 10.1289/ehp.1307277.

72. Alexeeff S, Litonjua A, Suh H, et al. Ozone exposure and lung function effect modified by obesity and airways hyperresponsiveness in the VA Normative Aging Study. Chest 2007;132(6):1890–7.

73. Lu K, Breysse P, Diette G, et al. Being overweight increases susceptibility to indoor pollutants among urban children with asthma. J Allergy Clin Immunol 2013; 131(4):1017–23.

74. Dong G, Qian Z, Liu M, et al. Obesity enhanced respiratory health effects of ambient air pollution in Chinese children: the Seven Northeastern Cities study. Int J Obes 2013;37(1):94–100.

75. Bennett W, Hazucha M, Folinsbee L, et al. Acute pulmonary function response to ozone in young adults as a function of body mass index. Inhal Toxicol 2007;19: 1147–54.

76. Epstein T, Ryan P, LeMasters G, et al. Poor asthma control and exposure to traffic pollutants and obesity in older adults. Ann Allergy Asthma Immunol 2012;108(6):423–8.

77. Jung K, Perzanowski M, Rundle A, et al. Polycyclic aromatic hydrocarbon exposure, obesity and childhood asthma in an urban cohort. Environ Res 2014;128: 35–41.

78. Lin C, Lin C. Work of breathing and respiratory drive in obesity. Respirology 2012;17(3):402–11.

79. Naimark A, Cherniack R. Compliance of the respiratory system and its components in health and obesity. J Appl Physiol (1985) 1960;15(3):377–82.

80. King G, Brown N, Diba C, et al. The effects of body weight on airway calibre. Eur Respir J 2005;25:896–901.

81. Zerah F, Harf A, Perlemuter L, et al. Effects of obesity on respiratory resistance. Chest 1993;103:1470–6.

82. Shore S, Rivera-Sanchez Y, Schwartzman I, et al. Responses to ozone are increased in obese mice. J Appl Physiol (1985) 2003;95:938–45.

83. Graham D, Chamberlain M, Hutton L, et al. Inhaled particle deposition and body habitus. Br J Ind Med 1990;47(1):38–43.

84. Hersoug L, Linneberg A. The link between the epidemics of obesity and allergic diseases: does obesity induce decreased immune tolerance? Allergy 2007; 62(10):1205–13.

85. Madrigano J, Baccarelli A, Wright R, et al. Air pollution, obesity, genes and cellular adhesion molecules. Occup Environ Med 2010;67(5):312–7.

86. Lang J, Williams E, Mizgerd J, et al. Effect of obesity on pulmonary inflammation induced by acute ozone exposure: role of interleukin-6. Am J Physiol Lung Cell Mol Physiol 2008;294(5):L1013–20.

87. Johnston R, Schwartzman I, Shore S. Macrophage inflammatory protein-2 levels are associated with changes in serum leptin concentrations following ozone-induced airway inflammation. Chest 2003;123(3 Suppl):369S–70S.
88. Dandona P, Aljada A, Bandyopadhyay A. Inflammation: the link between insulin resistance, obesity and diabetes. Trends Immunol 2004;25(1):4–7.
89. Schikowski T, Schaffner E, Phuleria H, et al. Improved air quality and attenuated lung function decline: modification by obesity in the SAPALDIA cohort. Environ Health Perspect 2013;121(9):1034.

Index

Note: Page numbers of article titles are in **boldface** type.

A

Adenosine monophosphate-activated protein, 810–812
Adipocytes
    environmental pollutants affecting, 839–849
    proinflammatory properties of, 848
Adipokines, 742, 758–759
Adiponectin, 758–759
Air pollution, obesity related to, **839–855**
    autonomic nervous system and, 846–847
    endocrine aspects of, 846–847
    epidemiology of, 841–842
    inflammatory pathway, 845–846
    mechanism of, 842–845
    polyaromatic hydrocarbons, 845
    vulnerability, 847–849
Airway hyper-responsiveness, 760
Allergy, in pediatric patients, 753–757
Antioxidants, 791, 829
Arginine metabolism, **767–775**, 791, 814–815
Arginine methyltransferase inhibitors, 768
Asthma
    epidemiology of, 740, 778–779
    epigenetics and, 826–828
    mitochondrial dysfunction in, 789
    obesity-associated, 758
        arginine metabolism and, **767–775**, 791, 811, 814–815
        bioenergetics of, **785–796**
        cause and effect relationship in, 755–758
        clinical features of, 743–744
        comorbid conditions in, 761, 803–804
        early-onset obesity associated, 743
        environmental pollution and, **839–855**
        epidemiology of, 739–741, 753–754
        epigenetic programming in, **825–837**
        in children, **753–765, 777–784**
        late-onset obesity associated, 744
        outcomes of, 744, 760–761
        pathophysiology of, 742, 758–760
        phenotypes of, **739–751**
        risk factors for, 740–741
        risk of, 754–755

Immunol Allergy Clin N Am 34 (2014) 857–862
http://dx.doi.org/10.1016/S0889-8561(14)00097-6
0889-8561/14/$ – see front matter © 2014 Elsevier Inc. All rights reserved.
immunology.theclinics.com

United States Postal Service

Statement of Ownership, Management, and Circulation
(All Periodicals Publications Except Requestor Publications)

1. Publication Title	2. Publication Number	3. Filing Date
Immunology and Allergy Clinics of North America	0 0 6 - 3 6 1	9/14/14

4. Issue Frequency	5. Number of Issues Published Annually	6. Annual Subscription Price
Feb, May, Aug, Nov	4	$320.00

7. Complete Mailing Address of Known Office of Publication (Not printer) (Street, city, county, state, and ZIP+4®)

Elsevier Inc.
360 Park Avenue South
New York, NY 10010-1710

Contact Person
Stephen R. Bushing

Telephone (Include area code)
215-239-3688

8. Complete Mailing Address of Headquarters or General Business Office of Publisher (Not printer)

Elsevier Inc., 360 Park Avenue South, New York, NY 10010-1710

9. Full Names and Complete Mailing Addresses of Publisher, Editor, and Managing Editor (Do not leave blank)

Publisher (Name and complete mailing address)

Linda Belfus, Elsevier Inc., 1600 John F. Kennedy Blvd., Suite 1800, Philadelphia, PA 19103-2899

Editor (Name and complete mailing address)

Jessica McCool, Elsevier Inc., 1600 John F. Kennedy Blvd., Suite 1800, Philadelphia, PA 19103-2899

Managing Editor (Name and complete mailing address)

Adrianne Brigido, Elsevier Inc., 1600 John F. Kennedy Blvd., Suite 1800, Philadelphia, PA 19103-2899

10. Owner (Do not leave blank. If the publication is owned by a corporation, give the name and address of the corporation immediately followed by the names and addresses of all stockholders owning or holding 1 percent or more of the total amount of stock. If not owned by a corporation, give the names and addresses of the individual owners. If owned by a partnership or other unincorporated firm, give its name and address as well as those of each individual owner. If the publication is published by a nonprofit organization, give its name and address.)

Full Name	Complete Mailing Address
Wholly owned subsidiary of	1600 John F. Kennedy Blvd, Ste. 1800
Reed/Elsevier, US holdings	Philadelphia, PA 19103-2899

11. Known Bondholders, Mortgagees, and Other Security Holders Owning or Holding 1 Percent or More of Total Amount of Bonds, Mortgages, or Other Securities. If none, check box ☐ None

Full Name	Complete Mailing Address
N/A	

12. Tax Status (For completion by nonprofit organizations authorized to mail at nonprofit rates) (Check one)
The purpose, function, and nonprofit status of this organization and the exempt status for federal income tax purposes:
☐ Has Not Changed During Preceding 12 Months
☐ Has Changed During Preceding 12 Months (Publisher must submit explanation of change with this statement)

PS Form 3526, August 2012 (Page 1 of 3 (Instructions Page 3)) PSN 7530-01-000-9931 PRIVACY NOTICE: See our Privacy policy in www.usps.com

---

13. Publication Title	14. Issue Date for Circulation Data Below
Immunology and Allergy Clinics of North America	August 2014

15. Extent and Nature of Circulation		Average No. Copies Each Issue During Preceding 12 Months	No. Copies of Single Issue Published Nearest to Filing Date
a. Total Number of Copies (Net press run)		426	492
b. Paid Circulation (By Mail and Outside the Mail)	(1) Mailed Outside-County Paid Subscriptions Stated on PS Form 3541. (Include paid distribution above nominal rate, advertiser's proof copies, and exchange copies)	256	263
	(2) Mailed In-County Paid Subscriptions Stated on PS Form 3541. (Include paid distribution above nominal rate, advertiser's proof copies, and exchange copies)		
	(3) Paid Distribution Outside the Mails Including Sales Through Dealers and Carriers, Street Vendors, Counter Sales, and Other Paid Distribution Outside USPS®	45	54
	(4) Paid Distribution by Other Classes Mailed Through the USPS (e.g. First-Class Mail®)		
c. Total Paid Distribution (Sum of 15b (1), (2), (3), and (4))		301	317
d. Free or Nominal Rate Distribution (By Mail and Outside the Mail)	(1) Free or Nominal Rate Outside-County Copies Included on PS Form 3541	60	100
	(2) Free or Nominal Rate In-County Copies Included on PS Form 3541.		
	(3) Free or Nominal Rate Copies Mailed at Other Classes Through the USPS (e.g. First-Class Mail)		
	(4) Free or Nominal Rate Distribution Outside the Mail (Carriers or other means)		
e. Total Free or Nominal Rate Distribution (Sum of 15d (1), (2), (3) and (4))		60	100
f. Total Distribution (Sum of 15c and 15e)		361	417
g. Copies not Distributed (See instructions to publishers #4 (page #3))		65	75
h. Total (Sum of 15f and g)		426	492
i. Percent Paid (15c divided by 15f times 100)		83.38%	76.02%

16. Total circulation includes electronic copies. Report circulation on PS Form 3526-X worksheet.

17. Publication of Statement of Ownership
If the publication is a general publication, publication of this statement is required. Will be printed in the November 2014 issue of this publication.

18. Signature and Title of Editor, Publisher, Business Manager, or Owner

Stephen R. Bushing

Date
September 14, 2014

Stephen R. Bushing – Inventory Distribution Coordinator
I certify that all information furnished on this form is true and complete. I understand that anyone who furnishes false or misleading information on this form or who omits material or information requested on the form may be subject to criminal sanctions (including fines and imprisonment) and/or civil sanctions (including civil penalties).

PS Form 3526, August 2012 (Page 2 of 3)

Printed and bound by CPI Group (UK) Ltd, Croydon, CR0 4YY

03/10/2024

01040491-0014